About the Author

Michael Saunders is a retired consultant neurologist and Anglican priest. He spent many years in both roles simultaneously and has worked predominantly in North East England and North Yorkshire. He spent a short time as a medical missionary in South India before returning to the UK through ill health. He is married to a consultant psychiatrist and has four adult children. He has muscular dystrophy and is a full-time wheelchair user.

From Certainty to Mystery

Michael Saunders

From Certainty to Mystery

Olympia Publishers
London

www.olympiapublishers.com
OLYMPIA PAPERBACK EDITION

A CIP catalogue record for this title is
available from the British Library.

ISBN: 978-1-78830-201-2

First Published in 2019

Olympia Publishers
60 Cannon Street
London
EC4N 6NP
Printed in Great Britain

Dedication

To Rene for her love and loyalty

Acknowledgments

I wish to acknowledge the many anonymous people who have been my patients and challenged and inspired me through my own struggles with disease. Without them this book would not have been written. I would like to thank also, those who have enabled me to reflect on the great faiths of our world. I would particularly wish to thank Peter Bishop, whose own journey has helped me to understand how it is possible to live within the religion of one's own culture while accepting and benefitting from the wisdom of other faiths.

Contents Page

Preface

During our lives most of us spend much of our time working in the secular world, at home and in the various environments where we earn our income. I refer to home because the life of the family requires work and commitment of fundamental importance. If we are of a religious disposition and belong to a specific religious framework we may pause, if we have time, to reflect on the interaction between our various roles in society and the faith we have followed. This may result in developments that surprise us. We may discover that the tightly knit faith structures that we grew up with require significant modification as a result of life experiences that impact profoundly on our world view. I have worked in the British National Health Service (NHS) my entire working life. When I was in my mid-forties I was ordained priest in the Anglican Church. I retained my normal NHS job as a consultant neurologist, thus becoming a minister in secular employment. By that time I was disabled by a progressive muscle disease. These three aspects of my life have interacted and resulted in considerable changes to my understanding of the faith structure I inherited. This book is about that interaction. I am in old age now and retired. This allows more time to think, but perhaps with a certain loss of clarity that besets most of us when the brain atrophies!

I have become convinced that all religions require secular academic study. This is not to deny the world of 'faith', but I do not see how one can live in the modern Western world without a thorough evaluation of religious claims. Globalisation has forced open minded people to reconsider the exclusivism of any religion. Two broad forms of Christianity have become apparent in recent years; the first I will call traditional Christianity, and the second, progressive Christianity. Orthodox views tend to be literalistic, exclusive, and have significant preoccupation with the afterlife. Progressive Christianity places emphasis on openness and exploration, absorbing the findings of science, including neuroscience, and the need to acknowledge the religious traditions of other great cultures. It is undogmatic and the word seeking rather than believing is appropriate. These two versions have led to conflict within the church. There is some overlap, but I have separated them to expose fundamental differences in understanding. In some situations the progressive Christian may feel more compatibility with an agnostic than a conservative Christian. The reader will learn how I have moved from one version to the other.

As a student in the conservative evangelical tradition of Christianity I was advised that a critical study of scripture and any other aspect of religious studies, for example Christian origins, could undermine my faith. I found this very unsettling. If one is seeking greater understanding, the rigours associated with any academic study must be a good thing. But it took some time to develop an attitude and approach that treated the substrate of my faith like any other academic subject. When I did, the result was both liberating and troubling.

The medical world has changed a good deal since I qualified as a doctor and my understanding of Christianity has had to change also. This does not surprise me now and I know that I cannot go backwards.

What I write is not academic but is more about issues in life that occur and interact one with another. The starting points vary considerably. Because there are three main strands to consider, the reader will find medical material, aspects of religion, and issues resulting from a chronic progressive disease. The various interactions are not included in all essays. Those concerned with my personal ill health predominate in early essays. Later ones are more concerned with some interaction between medicine and religion, even if the latter is not always explicitly elaborated.

Although my approach to orthodox Christianity is critical, it is not possible to criticise peaceful religious faith. Genuine faith is a source of comfort to others, and in the brief cameos I supply of other people in their struggles, I do not denigrate what they believe unless they insist that theirs is the only way.

The conflict within Christianity has caused some progressive Christians to leave the Church. I have no wish to do that. I have found many people receptive to new ways of understanding their faith; and some of those outside the formal Church have been encouraged to join, in the hope they will be accepted as seekers rather than believers. What is a Christian? That remains the central debate; the answer may determine the future of the Church.

Introduction

It is self-evident that our world is full of differing beliefs and faiths. Some have a structure that allows them to fall into the definition of a religion, although the definition of what constitutes a religion may not be agreed universally. To avoid undue discussion of this it is agreed, generally, that Judaism, Christianity and Islam are religions. Hinduism is a religion, although less tightly structured than the religions of the Book. I regard Buddhism as a religion, although some might not, and understand it more as a way of living. Apart from formal religion there are many beliefs that reflect unstructured faith in miracles, the power of nature, and the importance of star signs and so on.

Within the broad gamut of complementary medicine, one might conclude that some kinds of treatment are more to do with beliefs than science. Despite our dependence on the products of scientific progress, many remain cynical and suspicious of all forms of science, including medical science.

Whatever our religion or set of beliefs, articulated or not, we can either test them against the world of our experiences and those of others, or choose to keep our beliefs independent of this kind of interaction. For most of us there is probably some kind of compromise and we are never as brutal with the painful consequences of honest interaction as we might be. This is unfortunate in a world that has changed so radically since the origin of the main religions. Yet, realism demands that we accept the numerous world views that exist on this Earth, however they are derived. A uniform world view seems an unlikely prospect. Civilisations and cultures have taken many different courses and religion has been at the heart of our cultural diversity. Cultures are an evolving dynamic phenomenon. Religions such as Christianity and Islam have spread through conquest and colonialisation. Africa and South America epitomise this. Where there has been a long established culture with sacred literature, Christianity has had less influence. The impact of Islam on India resulted from initial conquest, followed by the establishment of a rich culture, predominantly in the North; this has become part of the history of that area. This book connects predominantly with Christianity, but refers to other faiths, particularly Hinduism.

It can only be about one individual's journey within Christianity. But it does represent a viewpoint that increasingly seeks to be heard. This is for a progressive understanding of Christianity and indeed other religions. Rather than abandon formal religion altogether many people long to see more honest debate about some of the doctrines of faith, enshrined in ancient literature, that have come to represent the core of orthodoxy. Heterodox beliefs have always existed. Sometimes, there have been rigorous attempts to suppress them; for example, the writings of Irenaeus against Gnosticism, a mixture of many understandings of the significance of Jesus and his nature. These are a diatribe against heterodox views at the end of the second century Common Era.

The one thing I have become aware of in my thinking, reading and experience is that none of us are consistent in our ideas and utterances about religious faith. We contradict ourselves all the time. The idea that there is a coherent systematic theology has never appealed to me after my early experiences. Therefore, I may well contradict myself at several points. I have wondered for a long time about the purpose of religion and whether it has any purpose in this life. The core of religion is mystery; mystery provides no knowledge of why we exist. The recognition that there is a ground of our being that is holy and sacred may lead us to worship that which we may call God, but how we live our lives depends on our own valuation as to what kind of life provides meaning and purpose for us. For the Christian, a decision has been made to follow the example of Jesus. This provides the meaning and purpose we seek. One conclusion for anyone who reflects about their religious faith against the background of experience is that if religion is to have any purpose, it does need to relate to daily living, and not be divorced from our lives. This means that the example of Jesus has to be translated into our current world. How we work this out will differ.

Although some of what I write may seem negative about religion I do want to emphasise that despite any appearances to the contrary, I remain positive about the importance of a religious framework to my life and those of others. The major task for a Christian is how Christianity can remain a viable faith in the Western world alongside the scientific progress and increased knowledge that has changed our lives.

I have selected a number of topics to write about. I could have chosen others, but these are some of the issues I have lived with. Some essays explore the difficulties with Christianity that I have experienced. Many essays are certainly autobiographical. They contain a good deal of personal material that I have placed in italics. Much of this is concerned with my experience of disease and disability. I did not think I could withhold it as it is a crucial part of me. It is not particularly easy to write about oneself, but I have come to the view that we all need to speak and write from experience. I refer also to the anonymous experiences of patients with whom I have shared my life.

Some of the chapter titles have an immediate religious element to them like the opening chapter on a child praying. There is a chapter named *Resurrection;* others have titles connected with disability such as *Falling* and *Weakness* and there are two on aspects of *Disability*. Later chapters have more general headings. They represent a kaleidoscope of topics that one might reflect on during the kind of life I have lived. Some may appear to have relatively little religious content. I write from the perspective that all aspects of life are sacred, whether or not we make specific references to religion.

Most of my previous written work has been in the field of neurology or medical ethics, but I have felt that the relatively unusual combination of priesthood, medicine and long-term disability in one person justifies the effort.

One of the greatest improvements in science has been the advent of multidisciplinary activity in solving problems. The approach to religion must be multidisciplinary. Failure to interact with what goes on in the world make it irrelevant. We must not practice our faith in a vacuum. But this is not a text book of medicine.

I am a founder member of the Society of Ordained Scientists and I continue to believe that there can be fruitful interaction between religion and science. Modern medicine is a scientific subject. One important feature that characterises scientific knowledge is that it is always provisional. We must be prepared to modify what we think and believe to be the case when new knowledge and discoveries become available. A simple example from my own speciality is the classification of muscular dystrophy. Until the emergence of modern molecular genetics, muscular dystrophy was classified according to clinical presentation, biochemical abnormalities and muscle biopsy. The advent of molecular genetics has made it evident that some of the dividing lines in earlier classifications were misplaced. It is becoming possible to reclassify these diseases based on the precise genetic defect and the abnormality that this gives rise to in structure and function.

I have developed the view that a similar process should apply in our dogmatic formulations. Dogma is an *attempt* to give structure and shape to experience. Any dogmatic structure should be expressed in the thought forms of a specific historical culture. The challenge for any great religion is how to express living experience in the light of current knowledge. This is a very difficult task for a dogmatic religion like Christianity, partly because there is an inbuilt resistance to radical reformulations; perhaps largely based on fear of the consequences. Those in authority in any great religion may be over concerned that the fabric of the institution they serve may crumble if the impact of any challenge to doctrine is acknowledged; but making doctrine that connects with our lives remains the ultimate issue, because most of us need some structure to live by.

I do not think that we should be looking for detailed parallels between science and religion. The idea that the one can prove the other is barren. What is important for the theologian and the scientist is to accept the provisional nature of all that we think and do and leave the door open for revision and change. Although some Christians would point to the absolute status of revelation, a word that is difficult to define, this does not imply an inability to change and modify. The Church has changed over the centuries because of knowledge that can be interpreted as revelation. Overall, the Church reacts after new human knowledge has been present for some time. It now faces difficulties because of the rapidity of scientific and technological progress and the globalisation of human knowledge and culture.

Marcel Proust's novel *Finding Time Again,* the final volume of *In Search of Lost Time*, contains insights to reflect on. In this novel Proust describes the search for the heart of any experience. At times, one may be struck very forcibly by something that happens, but at other times we struggle to isolate the essence of our lives. We can go through life with very little insight because we spend little time below the surface of our personal narrative. Beyond the time structured story we struggle to touch the mystery of our existence. Although our lives are mundane much of the time, occasionally we are caught unawares and our understanding is illuminated for a moment, a glimpse of something beyond ourselves, eternal and treasured.

The reader will find some repetitions in the book. There are reasons for this. The primary features of religion are concerned with relatively few issues. We are preoccupied with death, the afterlife, the action or otherwise of God in the world, the problem of evil, the impact of the various prophets and saviours, and the question of why we are here and how we should live. Starting from a certain point, reflection may readily take one in the same direction as other journeys. As each chapter is to some extent independent repetition can be helpful. Examples of this are references to soul and spirit in several chapters.

I have attempted to use language that is readily understood and to explain technical terms used. There are plenty of clinical histories that are part of my experience as a doctor. These stories are anonymous but real.

This book is intended for those with or without a specific religious affiliation. It may be read by those who have a general interest in disease and disability. I hope it will appeal to a wide readership as it contains the kind of material that connects with us all as we pass through life. Although it is written from a Western Christian viewpoint it is written with respect for other traditions and all faiths. Any biblical quotations are from the New International Version, Anglicised edition. I have used the notations Before Common Era (BCE) and Common Era (CE) as they reflect the neutrality necessary in a diverse world. I have referred to the Old Testament, and occasionally used the term Hebrew Bible (Tanakh). Although the two differ in some content and arrangement it is essential that Christians acknowledge that their faith stems from Judaism. I regret that I have referred to God as He on occasions because of grammatical issues, but fully acknowledge that God has no gender.

I have provided a limited list of books and papers for further reading.

A Child's Prayer

"Then you will call on the name of your God, and I will call on the name of the Lord. The God who answers by fire – he is God."
I Kings 18.24

"Prayer is not asking. It is a longing of the soul. It is daily admission of one's weakness. It is better in prayer to have a heart without words than words without a heart."
Mahatma Gandhi

The small boy rose from his knees and looked in the mirror. One or other eye was still in the corner of the socket. One eye would stay central, the other would deviate outwards, the pupil and iris disappearing into the corner of the globe. This would precipitate the remark from people: 'Where are you looking?'

There was no improvement. The prayer had been one of a series of varying intensity and duration. The results had always been negative.

The resort to prayer was one line of treatment for an intractable alternating external squint that had begun to trouble him. There had been a visit to an ophthalmologist who recommended nothing apart from a series of orthoptic exercises that did not help. Subsequently, an alternative therapist had suggested that repeated bathing of the eyes in cold water would strengthen the eye muscles. There followed a series of trials of varying length and intensity, rather like the prayers and equally unsuccessful.

Looking back on this childhood experience I am aware of the temptation to over-elaborate what I can remember. I was certainly upset by all the treatment failure and aware that I had a genuine physical problem. I do not know what I thought about God at that time. I accepted the prayer failure and I am not aware that I thought this diminished the importance or credibility of God. I certainly do not recall this as a trial like the famous battle by fire between Elijah and the prophets of Baal. But children are very practical and my main concern was whether prayer worked or not in achieving a specific end. It was self-evident that prayer for one's own benefit was suspect! At least it did not work with this god, and I was unaware of any other. If I had enquired further, I would have realised the conflict between the texts I had heard about asking and receiving and my own negative experiences. It does seem perfectly natural when something bad happens to you to make a request to God to change it. This experience was the beginning of a long path concerning my understanding of the nature of prayer.

I found the wordiness of prayer a problem. I was living in a South Coast town and was taken by my parents with my brother and sister to a local tabernacle. Sometimes we would stay for the whole service instead of Sunday School. My main memory of these occasions was the endless stream of language during the long extemporary prayers and sermons. The minister spoke interminably in a loud impassioned voice. God was assaulted by words during the prayers. I cannot recall any silence. One of my reactions, other than boredom, was to burst into uncontrollable giggles that had to be stifled with a handkerchief.

Prayer was all about language, making requests, calling on God to do all kinds of things. Like many children I was taught to say my prayers, kneeling by my bed. These consisted of requests to God to take care of others in the family and those in need. I did not consciously appreciate the value of silence although I spent a good deal of time on my own, thinking.

During my life, I would have loved God to magic away the various physical diseases that I have developed. No one wants to go through life with chronic ill health. But I have never thought that it was part of God's role in creation to cure my physical ailments outside human knowledge and behaviour. There have been times, in acute distress, when I have prayed for relief in anger or emotional turmoil, but that is something that most people do regardless of their specific beliefs. Some years ago I was in hospital after an operation and was both upset and in severe pain. There was difficulty obtaining pain relief. I certainly cried out that I wanted God to help me. The real relief came with an injection of morphine.

Frequently, during my medical career, I have wanted people with incurable disease to become better. People with multiple sclerosis, malignant brain tumours, motor neurone disease, muscular dystrophy and many other conditions. It is not my experience that God works in the world in this way. If he exists and is abroad in his creation, he works through us in making things come right.

I recall a conversation I had some time ago with an ordinand. We were discussing healing. The ordinand was quite convinced that God can heal any physical abnormality, the missing ingredient for unsuccessful healing was lack of faith and prayer. I countered his argument using the example of the treatment of leprosy. I had had some experience of this in India. I pointed out that I had never seen God grow new noses or digits for those damaged by disease. I had seen outstanding work done in reconstructive surgery which resulted in considerable functional improvements. Early treatment of leprosy with new drugs has prevented much physical deformity.

This argument did not convince the ordinand. The experience of others from cultures and worlds alien to his own could not be absorbed. I have encountered similar attitudes on other occasions. Although there are numerous ways of understanding the world, I have always found this one difficult to feel tolerant about.

On a weekend course at a theological college some years ago I saw a notice requesting greater prayer effort for a well-known Anglican minister and evangelist. The notice stated he was getting worse and much more prayer effort was required. The picture created was of a god who was either deaf or needed a certain level of prayer volume to respond.

I do not wish to embark on a lengthy theological discourse, but personal experience of disease in me and others raises several basic questions about religion and theism.

It is possible to use language such as 'God answers prayer', but if this does not fit in with personal experience one should ask whether there is a god at all, and if there is, what kind of god exists? Orthodox theism depends on the notion of a personal god. Theism certainly separates Christianity, Judaism and Islam from Buddhism, despite any different emphases in the three religions of the Book.

It is the personal interaction between God and people that creates the problem, and the tendency to separate humans from other forms of life. A personal god is irrelevant in Buddhism. One does not need to bother about this issue. Humans are part of a whole, who can only attain their destiny by transcending suffering and seeking enlightenment in this world.

Belief in a personal god raises the question of theodicy and much time has been expended attempting to answer the philosophical question: 'How can a loving God allow evil and suffering?' In my opinion, it is unanswerable if one takes an orthodox view of theistic monotheism. Disease exists. Catastrophe exists. Those who wish to extrapolate from individual belief frameworks, centered around a belief that God looks after them and will prevent them from suffering, should build a system to explain the experiences of others less fortunate than themselves. I would suggest that it is easier to conclude that the world is a harsh place and that there is no convincing evidence that God has created a universe in which he intervenes in any obvious way. We are left to look after each other.

Many believers seem to be afraid of considering that God has limited himself in his creation. Creation is God but God is more than that. He is transcendent. This is panentheism as opposed to pantheism. Any risk in creating may be perceived as threatening the omnipotence of God. This is not the case. God can limit himself within his own nature, and if this is the best of all possible worlds or potentially the best of all possible worlds, there is no real threat to belief in God and his presence in the cosmos. If we do not accept as real, the nature of the world we live in, and expect God to alter it for our convenience, we can never live comfortably with ourselves or the experience of others.

Any doctor or nurse who spends a life working in a hospital lives with premature disease and death. Children and young adults develop conditions that cannot be cured with the current state of scientific knowledge, and die. People are born with genetic abnormalities that cause disease at various stages of life. This may be puzzling and distressing, but much of that puzzlement is governed by our own expectations. We project on to God what we expect of him. We project our own ideas of love, fairness, and so on.

We know that creation is not static. The world continues to change and evolve. In medicine, scientific knowledge develops and diseases become treatable; progress is made after years of arduous research and development. Then new diseases appear such as HIV infection. We are faced with a changing picture as creation unfolds. Human knowledge has eventually reached a point when we can begin to modify the creative process and take more and more control over our own destiny. One can argue that this means we have potentially become co-workers with God.

I have a genetic disease myself. It is a rare and slowly progressive form of muscular dystrophy. In my case the precise genetic abnormality is still unknown, but I keep in touch with my genetics consultant. I do not expect God to cure this condition without human effort. I have no difficulty now accepting that I have been unfortunate like many others, without impairing any awareness of the presence of a transcendent God imminent also in creation. I take the view that human endeavour will gradually result in the accumulation of sufficient scientific knowledge to allow prevention or treatment eventually. It is very unlikely that this will happen in my lifetime.

As mentioned, creation carries a huge risk, the potential for many things to go wrong. This applies to all creative activity whether it be giving birth, creating art, music, poetry. Creation is painful. It is costly. There is no creative possibility without risk. In an existence limited by the dimensions of space and time it is understandable that we are angry and puzzled by unmerited diseases and strange natural events such as earthquakes. We cannot understand how these episodes can be consistent with a loving and all-powerful god. We misunderstand the nature of creation. This is the problem of limited vision. We long for logical intellectually satisfying answers, but there are none. We may have a lot of knowledge but it is limited by the nature of our brains. We examine the world in one way.

Whether we make the leap of faith and believe in a loving God does seem to some extent to depend on whether we can cope with the idea that creatures cannot expect to know and understand everything. There is an ultimate mystery about ultimate truth.

At the end of the first edition of his book *A Brief History of Time* Stephen Hawking stated that if we knew a unifying theory to explain the material universe, we would know the mind of God. But any insightful doctrine of God presumes that God is unknowable and any such scientific understanding could never be knowledge of God, even if it was an intimation of God's creative activity.

The 'leap' of faith is illustrated by a well-known parable told by John Wisdom and quoted by Anthony Flew in *The Existence of God*, edited by John Hick.

The story is told of two people who enter a jungle clearing and debate whether amidst the tangle there is evidence of a gardener having visited. The sceptic denies it and after many observations concludes there to be no tangible evidence of a visitor. He sees a jungle with no evidence of design, a disordered tangle of foliage. The other sees things differently; for that person it is possible to believe that there is a gardener at work despite evidence to the contrary. The key to the parable is that both agree about the basic evidence before their eyes. One comes to one conclusion, the other another. The difference is not based on rational argument.

When there is no obvious answer to a prayer we may use the phrase: 'It was not God's will'. This allows us to keep faith with God through our acknowledging that we are unable to know fully His mind. Another will conclude that the whole idea of God is mistaken.

Because of the limitations and risks in creation I have described, there is a responsibility placed on us to use our time and talents to make a difference in this world. Some versions of religion encourage fatalism and passiveness. Somehow, we expect someone else to put things right. When we attempt to make a difference in this world others may be angry with us when we fail. In some way we identify with God in our failure; we share his pain and He/She shares ours. There is a reciprocity that hints at the true nature of prayer. If we reach this state our exasperation and anger with God falls away. We have begun to learn about listening to the heart beat of existence, rather than wanting God to do all the hearing.

Many people do claim that petitionary prayer 'works'. They remain comfortable with the idea of a listening God who *does* respond. There are numerous examples of dramatic healing of apparent severe disease. I intend to cover the topic of healing elsewhere. At this stage I would point out that there is a subtle difference between impairment and disability caused by specific pathological mechanisms and 'illnesses' of less certain aetiology. Even so, the level of impairment and disability can be profoundly affected by the overall state of the individual, their state of 'wholeness'. Petitionary prayer, if the person prayed for is aware of the prayers of others, may contribute to increased wellbeing.

I recall several experiences that help to focus the issue of petitionary prayer. I prayed very hard once for a young woman under my care with cancer of the breast together with a neurological problem known as polymyositis that resulted from the cancer. This caused generalised weakness of the muscles. She was married to a fireman and they had a young daughter. Yvonne had a job as a gardener. She deteriorated and developed difficulty breathing. She was admitted to hospital in a distressed condition. She did not recover and died a few days later. The one redeeming feature of her last days was that shortly before she died she became peaceful, the agony and the distress were laid aside. But I met her husband a year or two later in a pub and he was not at peace. The loss had shattered his life. This was a straightforward tragedy. I prayed initially that this young woman would be cured. The most that can be stated is that she was not in acute distress when she died. The subsequent meeting with her husband confirmed the fear that her death damaged him badly. Sadly, limited resources had been made available to help him cope with this terrible loss. It strikes me that many of our attitudes to petitionary prayer are an escape from reality. We find it very difficult to live with the suffering people experience. We want an easy solution. It was natural for me to pray for this sick lady because her condition moved and distressed me, yet in my heart, my experience of life had already told me that she would die.

Modern expectations and attitudes do not take easily to adversity. I sometimes look at burial plaques from the 19th century and earlier. Many children died young. The attitude to life expectancy was completely different. Modern medicine had not arrived.

There was a greater emphasis on the gift of life rather than length of life. Human physical suffering was a present reality. It was not possible to escape it, for it to be outside the normal experience. Support arrangements at times of loss were different. There was little professional expertise available. People were dependent on their own resources and immediate family and friends. There was little expectation that God answered prayer. The evidence of His absence was everywhere. Any compensation lay elsewhere.

A modern story concerns Peter. His father was dead. Peter developed a progressive curvature of the middle part of his spine known as a dorsal scoliosis. Investigation revealed that the cause was an intrinsic tumour in the substance of the spinal cord, termed an astrocytoma. Although it is now possible to operate on these tumours, at that time, most surgeons were very reluctant to do so. The tumour was very extensive. Treatment was given with radiotherapy. Peter became completely paralysed in the legs and was a wheelchair user. He was an able person and did well at school, enabling him to go on to further education. Peter and his mother were devout Roman Catholics. In the face of this profound sorrow that her only son was disabled just as he was approaching adult life, Peter's mother wrote to me to say how grateful they were to God for all that they had been given. There was no trace of bitterness and no destruction of the shared family faith. This was a deeply rooted pious trust in God and looking at the positive rather than the negative aspects of life.

I am uncertain that whatever is beyond the grave makes up for a life time of unmerited suffering, but in some instances the word 'suffering' implies that we are in a state of mind or attitude which concentrates on the negative rather than the positive. Although I have often found positive attitudes difficult to maintain in my own difficulties, the example of Peter, his mother and others like them have ministered to me. There was no expectation that prayer would cure the disease, but the experience that life could be transformed. The disease could not be denied. but there was hope that what lay ahead had meaning and purpose with God at the heart of it. I have found this type of response a clue to the deeper meaning of prayer that one eventually understands more as the years go by. As TS Eliot has intimated in the *Four Quartets*, prayer is not necessarily a conscious mental activity, it is rather an attitude towards God, creation and other people. It is more about stillness and openness than striving. However, we may well, in communal prayer and privately, lift people before God and give our all in trying to care for them and help them if it is appropriate.

A very different reaction was expressed to me initially by a middle-aged couple. The husband had developed a malignant brain tumour at the age of forty-eight. I sat down and told him the diagnosis and the likely outcome. He said he wanted to know as he was an executive in a large company and needed to take the appropriate actions. On hearing the news he was upset and his wife was very angry at my telling him. He refused all palliative care and left the hospital immediately. I never met him again as he refused to come and see me. I was very upset at the time and the circumstances lived in my memory, so that when I came across his wife in a neighbouring market town several years later I had no difficulty recognising her. She stopped me and we passed the time of day. She then said that she wanted to tell me that her husband had lived for six months and that it had been the most precious time in their lives together. They could share things with an intimacy that had not been there before. It would not have been possible if the diagnosis had not been shared. His death was tragic, but the initial anger had been transformed into something beautiful and eternal.

The couple were keen Christians. They had prayed that a cure would occur despite medical impotence. This did not happen, but their grief and anger were transformed into a relationship of sufficient beauty to defeat the limitations of time. They experienced a new quality of life, not previously found over many years of being together.

My childhood experience taught me an early lesson. Prayer is not a mechanical activity. There is nothing wrong in sharing the deep feelings of our hearts, but we live in a world of limitation that we need to accept. None of us can escape from the risks of creation; but we can transform our anxiety and grief through experiences of the eternal, reminding us that life is about quality rather than quantity. But I must admit that those words sound very complacent. I feel I cannot press this too far. The next chapter refers to an *Indian Interlude*. This provided my first experience in which the basic facts of human existence were so bad that it was difficult to see life at that extreme as anything more than a struggle for survival. The remarkable thing was that even in the worst environments of a city such as Kolkata there were glimpses of hope, even in the very worst of conditions. Fine sounding words can only have meaning on a global front when we truly care about what happens beyond our immediate world.

Some years elapsed before the small boy with the external alternating strabismus saw any improvement in the condition. By this time he was at a boarding school, approaching fifteen years and very self-conscious. A visit to the school doctor one day resulted in a referral letter to another ophthalmologist. The adolescent steamed open the envelope to see what it said. The letter was forthright and expressed the view that unless something was done significant psychological trauma would occur. The writer was doubtless aware of the rigours of single sex boarding school life!

Eventually, a consultation took place at a local eye hospital. The surgeon indicated that an operation was perfectly possible, but explained that it would be difficult to achieve a complete correction at one go, a second operation might be needed. He expressed considerable surprise that nothing had been done earlier. After an operation was performed in those days, bandages were placed over the eyes for several days after surgery. When they were removed, there was initial double vision, but the eyes were straighter. Although there have been other operations they were not performed for many years. Nevertheless, the improvement was something to feel ecstatic about. A huge burden had been removed. It was a partial cure, but more importantly it was a healing. He was in a heightened vulnerable emotional state at the time, but still remembers with great vividness that experience.

It was his first real encounter with a hospital. He was very aware of the caring attitude of the nurses. Although he could not articulate this at the time, nurses remained for him models of skilled loving care. Their knowledge and their presence with the patient through good and bad spoke more eloquently than any sermon he had ever heard. Other experiences over the years reinforced this initial response but none were as potent.

One hesitates to record that this was the reason why I became a doctor, but it was. Surely an adolescent experience cannot have had such impact? At the time I had no intention of pursuing a profession with scientific content. I was more interested in English and Classics. My father was in horticulture. My mother had been a nurse for a short while, but I never thought men could be nurses in those days! I felt completely ill-equipped to become a doctor, but the feeling that I should become one did not waver and I managed to obtain a place at a London medical school, without studying science. The first year was difficult and did little to assuage doubts about my ability to study medical subjects. When the results came out on the Senate House notice board I had to return to look again to make sure I had passed! It seems bizarre to think that the pattern of my life was so influenced by one experience, but I have no other explanation for why I studied medicine.

The other memorable result of the operation was the overwhelming sense of a new birth, a new beginning. I suppose this was symbolised by the removal of the bandages and the sudden rush of light after a period of darkness. The most vivid memory is the pattern of light through Sussex beech and oak, as my mother took me for drives through the countryside near home, or as I walked on my own. There have been a few other experiences of similar exultation, most of them in my case have been related to recovery from illness and are referred to elsewhere. One supposes the word 'joy' is an appropriate one to describe the timeless sense of being alive. One could also apply the word 'resurrection'.

This was the eventual outcome of the child's prayer. It laid a foundation for a down-to-earth approach to how God acts in the world.

An Indian Interlude

"God is a name for that ultimate Mystery when it is seen in
relation to man, as Creator, Lord, Saviour, or whatever it may
be. Of this God it is reasonable to ask whether he exists or not.
But of the Godhead, of the ultimate Truth, one cannot ask
whether it exists. It is the ground of all existence."
Bede Griffiths *Journey to the Centre*

*The young neurologist sat in his cubicle in the main outpatient
department. It was July. Overhead a fan whirred to make the
intense heat and humidity a little more tolerable. South India is
always hot and the early afternoon at Vellore near Madras
(Chennai) was more suited to a siesta than an outpatient clinic.
People did register for attendance and notes were available, but
the chaos outside the small room bore little resemblance to the
sanitised waiting area of a Western hospital*

*There was a stable type door separating the room from the
outside corridor. Usually, both the upper and lower parts of the
door were open. The room accommodated the doctor and
sometimes an assistant who doubled up as interpreter. Various
relatives accompanied the patient and spilled over into the
corridor, where the next in line and their relatives jostled to see
what was going on.*

*People came here from all over India. Relatives would carry
a sick family member by train for days, to seek a medical opinion.*

The languages spoken were unpredictable. Many local Tamil speaking patients came, but the language might be Telugu, Hindi, Bengali or one of the many different Indian languages. The neurologist could speak none of them, just a few words of Tamil gleaned from his long-suffering teacher.

The patient in the room had epilepsy. It would be necessary to arrange an electroencephalogram and prescribe some medication. Although phenobarbitone prescribing had fallen into decline in the West it was the simplest and cheapest drug to use in India and was widely available. There was no point in prescribing drugs that could not be paid for and were unavailable on any long-term basis. Even then, one had to decide whether the family could afford any fees charged. They would certainly claim extreme poverty. It was important to decide whether this was genuine, an impossible task for an inexperienced Englishman. Fortunately, Rajagopalan, the departmental secretary and a supreme guide in all such matters, would assist in the decision. The patient and family were sent on their way to see him.

The heat was oppressive, the neurologist felt fed up. He had been in India a month or two. Why was he here? What had driven him to come to India with his wife and two small children? Was it a ghastly mistake that they would all regret?

I was not happy. I realised that I had misjudged what I had to offer. I was learning a great deal. In a few short weeks, every facet of tuberculosis of the nervous system had come through the department. Such exposure would not be achieved in a lifetime in the United Kingdom. I saw leprosy, infestations, advanced cerebral tumours, and cerebral vascular disease in young people. The whole gamut of clinical neurology was there. The work was fascinating. I registered for a DM in neurology at Madras University. But I was unhappy about the political climate in the department and unsure of my role and myself.

Apart from the medical work, there was anxiety about the nature of mission. My experience of other cultures and other religions was very limited before our arrival at the Christian Medical College Vellore. I had read about Hinduism and Islam, but had never entered dialogue with people of other faiths. I had been educated to take an exclusive view of Christianity. This is an unpromising starting point when considering the value of other religions and cultures. Missionaries were meant to draw people to Christianity. It was not an option to accept the intrinsic value of a genuine spiritual journey in a different culture, within a different fiduciary framework.

The central question for me was the problem of letting go of reassuring certainties and examine the spiritual insights of another culture and religion, without pre-conceived conclusions. One might argue that this is an impossible task. It is, in part. We cannot entirely escape our own cultural conditioning. Such a leap is made much easier if we can accept the possibility that *'Truth is Two Eyed'*, the title of a book on interfaith dialogue by the late John Robinson. By this is meant that it is possible to live with the notion that there is more than one way to pursue a spiritual journey. No path is exclusively right or wrong. Absolute truth lies beyond all religions. They are human inventions inspired by an innate desire to explain our lives on earth and connect in some way with the absolute meaning of everything. At the beginning of this chapter I have quoted from the writings of Bede Griffiths. As a Benedictine monk, living in South India, he was much influenced by Hinduism. He came to realise that the structures of all religions, including their gods, prophets and saviours, are not the final answer to the question of the Godhead's existence. Truth lies beyond this. In India, I began to realise that this was something I had to pursue further. It was the beginning of a long journey.

Hinduism, has not, in general, had the problems with exclusivism shared by the Judaeo-Christian tradition and Islam. But one must admit that recent events on the Indian sub-continent challenge this opinion. Despite this, Hindus tend to be much more tolerant of other ways and the many traditions within Hinduism. Christianity has yet to face realistically the exclusivist position arising from 'orthodox' Christian doctrine. The life and work of Jesus is a problem for Christians epitomised in the words:

"I am the way, the truth and the life. No one comes to the Father except through me." John 14.6.

I suppose how we read a text like this depends entirely on our view of John's Gospel and scripture in general. It provides a useful example of how the Bible divides Christians. Movements, such as the Jesus Seminar, do not consider that many if any of the words of the Gospels and particularly John's Gospel were spoken by Jesus. The latter is a theological work by a writer that presents Jesus as the pre-existent Logos or Word. He is identified with Sophia or Wisdom. To many the Jesus of John may appear as a weird and unearthly figure. John's Gospel was accepted into the Christian canon at a late stage, probably because of its susceptibility to Gnostic interpretation. It is not, in my view, a reliable guide to Jesus' thinking. Regardless of what this text might mean, real dialogue should include the possibility that God is revealed in other ways. Incarnation might not be exclusive to

Jesus. Jesus is a uniquely important figure for Christians, but he is not uniquely important for followers of other paths; although many religions honour Jesus, son of Mary.

The idea that God should be revealed exclusively in a historical context is truly remarkable. Jesus could be important to people of all faiths and cultures. But it began to seem a possibility that it was reasonable to follow the religion appropriate to one's own cultural background without rejecting or undermining the spiritual integrity of people of other faiths. If this was the case, it freed people to engage in non-threatening dialogue and share insights that would help them in their own spiritual journey, within their own religion. It was obvious to me that I could not become a Hindu, a Buddhist or a Muslim. I had no wish to do so. Perhaps, a few would be suited to cross the boundaries, but cultural considerations could not be ignored. Because there were such marked social and cultural differences between Indian and Western civilisations, the challenge was to avoid condemning one because of unfamiliarity.

I was encouraged from time to time by speaking to missionaries who had discovered the importance of dialogue. I recognised the need to talk and get to know people, without feeling under pressure to want to know what they believed.

Looking back from a more distant standpoint, I realise that I began to cease to trust some of the intellectual rigour of evangelical scholars, when defending or promoting exclusive pictures of Christianity. A whole series of questions began to appear. On the surface, they appeared threatening to one's own personal framework. Yet, they were essential for someone trained to think the unthinkable and I had been trained in one part of my life to question everything. The problem with many excellent scholars is that they operate within their field exclusively. This is not a problem in pure academic research that is unaffected by a personal world view, although multidisciplinary collaboration is vital in making scientific progress.

Isolated academic work is common in the study of religion. Although theology has a venerable place in the academic curriculum, it is perpetually in danger of being undermined by lack of objectivity. One reason for this that occupied me was the problem of failing to take note of other disciplines, particularly science. Some doctrines require the acceptance of happenings, described as historical, that have no rational explanation and challenge credulity in a world that has radically changed since their original development. Although some scientists are persuaded that the supernatural is possible, the very term is anathema to science. The word 'unexpected' is not. For example, modern medicine cannot explain the new life of a resurrected body or a new celestial body. If, in discussing the resurrection one is referring to a totally new Jesus who has undergone transformation, any literal interpretation of such an event is beyond ordinary human experience and has no scientific explanation.

Empiricism enters the world of religion, causing an obsession with literal reality. The worlds of logos, meaning scientific thinking and the need to have a faith couched in logos rather than mythos, is a disaster. The only way religion can survive is to return to metaphor and myth. Science challenges the logos of literal dogmatic claims.

The world of Indian religion was full of mythos and I realised that there was no pressure to take one view of Indian legends and sacred literature. There is no real clash between the mythos of Hinduism and science. There need be no clash between Christianity and science.

I was convinced after my sojourn in India that claims of Christian exclusivism did not add up. They were an insult to common sense. It would have been highly improbable that God would reveal himself so locally in one part of his creation. There might be differences in religious understanding across the planet, but the whole idea of a chosen people and a Man-God, who was the only source of salvation, did not add up.

The neurologist and his family sat drinking coffee and lemonade in a colleague's house at the medical college after morning service. He began to feel unwell, nauseated and feverish. He signalled to his wife that it was time to go and they made their excuses. They just managed to reach the flat before the vomiting started. The initial impression was that this was just another stomach upset and would settle soon enough, but there was no improvement. Fever, nausea and vomiting and abdominal pain continued. Jaundice was noticed. They assumed that this was just a brief bout of hepatitis that would settle, but a doctor was called. The provisional diagnosis was agreed; liver function tests showed a pattern consistent with infective hepatitis. The symptoms did not settle. Liver function deteriorated, the jaundice became more marked. Every time there was an attempt to get up vomiting restarted and liver function deteriorated. After several weeks he was admitted to a ward in the main hospital. By this time the spleen was greatly enlarged, extending into the left lower abdomen. No new diagnosis was made, but the expected improvement did not occur.

The room in the hospital was a single unit, a perk for being a staff member. It was pleasant and open to the outside air. There was a central ceiling fan. The main problem was the bats! They are wonderful creatures, but when they swooped in and out of the room over the bed, they lost some of their fascination. At times, it was necessary to lie with the sheet over his head.

Being in hospital, a long way from home in a strange country, is a challenging experience. It is made worse if one is aware of a level of concern and uncertainty amongst the staff; but the main problem in this case was severe homesickness, compounded by uncertainty surrounding the whole project of going to live in India. He never discussed this. He would lie in bed reading improving books about mission and wondering whether he was going to live or die. He thought of all the trouble he had caused his family. At other times, he dreamed of convalescence in the hills; he made plans, including the possibility of moving to Ludhiana, where there was an urgent need for a neurologist.

Initially, there was a general expectation that it would all settle down, but the jaundice persisted; there was no improvement in liver function, the spleen was very large.

Food was brought in from home in little containers, but he had no appetite. Friends visited and were very supportive. The local Church of South India minister came and gave him communion.

One day his wife came in with bad news. Their daughter had been playing in a sandpit in the hospital compound near the flat and been bitten by a stray dog. At the time, rabies was endemic in the town dog population and they strayed into the hospital grounds. The bite was on the chest. The incubation period for rabies is long, but it is related to the location of the bite, being longest the further it is away from the brain. Rabies is a universally fatal virus infection of the central nervous system; the only way to prevent it at that time was a protracted course of vaccination during the incubation period.

The dog had been caught. It was kept and clinical rabies confirmed. The young neurologist knew about rabies, but he was helpless to do much about it. He did not wish his daughter to have the older type of vaccine, with a high incidence of serious side effects, including vaccine damage to the nervous system. A duck embryo vaccine had been produced recently. None was available at Vellore, but there was a possibility that it was available at the American Embassy in Madras (Chennai). A car was sent to try and obtain it. On return, it was noted to be out of date, but better than nothing. Although the wound had been cleaned there was no immune serum to inject around it, another important aspect of rabies prevention at that time. It is easy to forget, with the development of the new safe vaccine, how difficult rabies immunisation used to be. There was no alternative but to start with injections of the out of date duck embryo vaccine into the anterior abdominal wall.

Christmas was approaching. Carol singers could be heard around the hospital. A week or two earlier, telegrams had been sent to hepatologists in London, asking for advice. Steroid drugs had been suggested. But the staff in Vellore were reluctant to use them.

The rabid dog bite was the turning point. Further telegrams were sent; a decision was made. His wife came to tell him they were being sent home. The feeling was one of dislocation and bewilderment.

On Christmas Eve, a van took them towards Chennai Airport. He lay on a stretcher in the back. They carried him on to the plane. He was laid across three seats. They took off from Chennai to Mumbai. He changed planes by being winched up on the food trolley.

London Airport on a cold Christmas morning seemed an alien world.

I have used the third person in describing some of my experience. The device may or may not work, but it helps to allow me to look at what happened. It may make reflection easier. The episode in India has required much thought over many years. I have had the opportunity to return to India as a doctor on several occasions and this has helped me to appreciate the wonder of this great country.

I suppose that several elements have emerged after reflection about this period of my life. From the health point of view, it was a turning point in my personal wellbeing. More importantly it provided me with a rapid exposure to clinical neurology and increased my experience dramatically. Both these medical aspects of my life have been very important. However, the most important lessons for me were cultural and spiritual.

I did not feel liberated at the time, but this was the beginning of a process of liberation that has excited me and given me peace that my narrow version of Christianity never achieved. Initially, I was a divided self, carrying on with my usual religious life, but inwardly attempting to work out a sustainable view of Christianity that could take account of other faiths and cultures. The main issue was related to the status of Jesus and the exclusive salvation claims connected with him.

The words of Bede Griffith at the beginning of this chapter seem to me to be fundamental in reformulating Christian dogma. 'The ground of our being', the goal of all religious quests, does not divide different religions. The many myths and stories that have entered specific religions have the potential to divide people, as they are developed from many different cultures. Globalisation, has increasingly exposed the divisive nature of exclusive religious claims that depend on a reliance on empiricism as opposed to mythological and metaphorical truth. The practical issue was and is the dilemma whether one can remain a Christian, within the framework of the institutional Church, or whether such an ideal is a lost cause. This remains an open question and it is a matter of personal judgement and current and future institutional attitudes. Some people become Church alumni because they no longer feel comfortable within the framework. Others soldier on, believing that for the Church to survive in the long term it is essential for people who adopt a pluralist view of religion to remain within their own faith. Increasingly, ordinary people who believe there is an ultimate source of their being, feel alienated by the demands of an organisation that appears to insist on the acceptance of specific doctrines, rather than a relaxed attitude to the content of individual belief.

Peter Bishop was my Church of South India minister and remains a close friend. He has written of the interaction of Christianity and other faiths in *Written on the Flyleaf – A Christian Faith in the Light of Other Faiths*. He concludes his book with the statement:

"The journey of faith may not after all provide the security we long for but are not granted in our complex, changing, bewildering world. It may do much more for us than that. As we make progress in our religious quest, we may find ourselves, to our surprise, exploring new scenery, crossing cultural boundaries, and as a result waking up to new ways of believing and practising our faith."

Wilfred Cantrell Smith, writing in *The Faith of Other Men*, made it clear that any serious doctrinal statement about Christianity had to explain the existence of great works like the Bhagavad Gita, and the fact that it exists and is a guide to many people.

Religious pluralism is something that bothers many sincere Christians. Yet we ignore the great historical religious traditions of other cultures at our peril. Alan Race, in *Christianity and Religious Pluralism*, points to arrogance and theological naiveté that underpin the assumption that only Christians apprehend religious truth. He referred to the theologian Paul Tillich. Tillich pointed out that at the core of all great religions, there is a point when the detailed framework of that religion falls away and loses its importance, and the disciple acquires a spiritual freedom that enables him/her to appreciate and adopt the many spiritual insights concerning the world and human existence

The point made by all these writers is that it is possible to live with integrity as a Christian or adherent of another great religion, but acknowledge the validity of other faiths within other cultures. Christianity has much to offer other traditions, but the traffic is not one way.

Weakness

"He was crucified in weakness, yet he lives by God's power."
2 Corinthians 13.4

"My grace is sufficient for you, for my power is made perfect in weakness."
2 Corinthians 12.9

The paradoxical idea that weakness can be a source of strength does not readily gain credence. In the animal kingdom, strength is linked with survival, weakness with death and loss of status. The survival of the fittest appears to be self-evident.

In human existence, it is obvious that weakness is a similar disadvantage. It would be unrealistic to think otherwise. However, for humans it is more likely that high intelligence will influence survival. The success of humanity is linked to intelligence rather than brute strength. Yet, it is undeniable that physical weakness is debilitating and a social disadvantage.

The Christian gospel thrives on paradox. It suggests to us that spiritual life and strength are not to be equated with physical and intellectual prowess. Strength may be associated with a feeling of physical invincibility. High intellect may be associated with sufficient arrogance to consider that any problem can be solved and there is nothing that cannot be explained and controlled. It is easy enough to see the grave spiritual dangers inherent in power and strength whatever the type. Any true spiritual life demands an acceptance of values beyond the achievements of physique, intellect and worldly power.

Weakness is an important symbol of human vulnerability, but the weakness of disease can never be good. However, it does point to the universal imperfection of all creation and the finitude of individual existence.

Sam and Tom were now teenagers. They came into the consulting room in electric wheelchairs with one hand still able to manoeuvre the controls. They seemed content as usual. I had never really seen them complain or appear miserable. This used to puzzle me. Mother always came with them. They seemed quite happy for her to be there. They never asked for a talk on their own. I went through the usual checks; wheelchair seating, straightness of the spine, cardiac status and a general review of care arrangements in the home.

Sam was two years older than Tom. They had both seemed normal at birth and had walked for a short period of their lives. It soon became obvious that they both had progressive weakness of the limbs and trunk. Initially, they had a laboured waddling gait; they climbed up themselves when standing up from the floor or a sitting position. The shoulder girdles were very weak. There was 'winging' of the shoulder blades.

When I first met them there was no difficulty coming to a rapid diagnosis. Apart from the clinical picture of progressive weakness in two young boys, investigations confirmed the diagnosis. Needle neurophysiology examination of the muscles revealed a primary muscle disease. The blood enzyme creatine kinase, released from damaged muscle, was greatly elevated. A muscle biopsy showed appearances typical of Duchenne

Muscular Dystrophy. The disease is carried on the female sex chromosome. The male has only one X chromosome and the disease is manifest if the X chromosome is abnormal. The mother carries the disease, but shows no clinical evidence of weakness. The only abnormality is a raised creatine kinase level in some carriers and minor changes on the other laboratory tests. The description for the mode of inheritance is a sex linked recessive disease. It has been shown in recent years that the disorder is linked with a severe deficiency of a muscle protein that has been named dystrophin. There is no cure currently.

Sam and Tom were wheelchair users before the age of ten. They became progressively weaker and were dependent for most acts of daily living. Boys with muscular dystrophy may live until the mid-twenties and usually die of heart disease or respiratory failure. Sam and Tom died in their early twenties.

The point of this description is to focus on an example of severe weakness.

Weakness has been a core element in my professional life, or rather the diagnosis and management of the many causes of this symptom. Weakness may develop suddenly or gradually. It may result from disease of the central nervous system, peripheral nerves, junction between nerve and muscle or the muscles. This story is about muscular dystrophy, a group of disorders, genetically determined, which produce progressive wasting and weakness of muscle. The age of onset, clinical course and pattern of weakness varies. The best-known type is Duchenne Muscular Dystrophy. Other varieties affect both sexes and may progress slowly over many years. Although there is no cure for muscular dystrophy, genetic research is making rapid progress in identifying the specific gene defect in many instances.

It was a Sunday morning. Instead of going to church he decided to have a rest and read the paper. As usual he turned to the sports pages. On the back of the section was an article on physical fitness. It involved a chart for guidance on self-examination. It is difficult to know what triggered his attempt at this. Perhaps it was those episodes of falling in the street. He had put it down to lack of physical fitness, never recovered after the spell in India. After a preliminary look at the lower limbs, he was very concerned. There was marked weakness of the thighs, particularly the quadriceps muscles and the glutei. He used a tendon hammer to examine his own reflexes and could not obtain them. In a panic he called his wife to confirm the findings, which she did. He had a disease, a neurological disease. This could not be due to simply being unfit.

At that time he was quite unable to reflect and bring into focus the many episodes that made sense of the findings. He had no clear diagnostic formulation in his mind. In his panic he telephoned his immediate colleague who kindly agreed to see him. A preliminary examination focused on the legs, confirmed the findings. Some preliminary neurophysiology was done and this seemed to raise the possibility of abnormal fatigability, a feature of a disorder known as myasthenia gravis. This is due to a defect in neuro-muscular transmission.

It was important to see someone more detached and he arranged to go and see a colleague at his former hospital.

One of the keys to accurate diagnosis in any branch of medicine is the history of the presenting complaint. The physician is like a detective, charting his/her way to the cause of the 'crime', eliciting information, asking the right questions, producing a hypothesis for subsequent confirmation or refutation. The history taker needs to get the best out of his/her subject and the limitations of time require the art to be highly developed for successful clinical practice. Doctors may blame the patient for providing inadequate or misleading information, but the fault may more often lie with lack of empathy, or inability to think with sufficient flexibility on the part of the doctor. The art of the history taker is against the background of detailed medical knowledge, a corpus of facts about diseases, and the many modes of presentation. I accept that modern imaging techniques have diminished the need for obsessive clinical examination, but it is those skills that I valued and remember. There is an attempt to ask three questions. Where is the problem, that is what part of the nervous system is involved? The condition may be in one specific anatomical site or the conclusion may be that it is a diffuse or multi-focal disorder. The second question is a consideration of possible causes, followed by an assessment of useful further investigations. Finally, there is the question of treatment, prognosis and support.

The journey to the hospital only confirmed that there was a real problem. A car tyre punctured; he did not have the strength in arms or legs to change it and became stuck on the ground, unable to stand up on a motorway hard shoulder. A passing police car came to his assistance.

He gave a poor history because he was unaware of the significance of various life events. The attention was on the legs and a link was made with the illness in India. It was thought he might have had a virus infection damaging the lower spinal nerve roots, but it was felt important to exclude spinal cord or nerve root compression due to a tumour. An investigation running radio-opaque dye up and down the spinal canal was arranged, a myelogram. The investigation was normal; some blood tests were performed. Several days later he had a telephone call. The blood creatine kinase was elevated. It was thought he must have some neuromuscular disorder. A paradigm shift in his understanding of his body took place; many things became clear. In what seemed a few minutes he went over his life.

When he was about ten years old he fell over and hurt his left arm. It was very painful, but he told nobody. He was afraid of medical exposure. Looking back, something made him think that not all was well. He had broken his right arm twice, but the problem that really worried him was a weakness in his arms he felt should not be there. They worked well enough generally, but he could not climb rope ladders or pull himself up on wall bars. He became terrified of gym lessons, of ridicule in front of other boys. He tried to strengthen his arms with a chest expander, but there was no change. The problem was not too intrusive as he could play cricket and football well for his age and won the school sprints.

Later, at boarding school, he was aware that sprint times were not improving, and boys he expected to beat overtook him. He managed with considerable effort to do well at cross-country until he was sixteen, but then his comparative performance fell away and he gave up running. He was puzzled, upset, but he told no one and asked for no advice. Until he was sixteen he had been good at football, agile with both feet and a striker in the under sixteen team; but performance deteriorated and he was dropped. He loved games and this was a bitter blow. He concentrated on less vigorous pursuits and played chess for the school.

At medical school he had attempted one game of football. He scored a goal with the stub of his toe. He was upset because he noticed he could hardly run. After the game he sat on the underground station and thought about it. He explained the problem by deciding he must have a bad knee; he had injured it once. Yet he did nothing about it; he did not go to a doctor. After all he had had a medical on arrival and had been told he was fit enough. There was no detailed examination and he had volunteered nothing, but he was able to live happily without thinking too much further. It was possible to adapt to slowly progressive weakness by changes in life style. He hid himself playing second team hockey, a little casual tennis and village cricket.

Life after qualification was hectic and there was little time to dwell on anything or take up hobbies that stressed the muscles. House jobs had no defined hours or off duty. He married on qualification and his wife, a doctor, worked in another hospital. They got together in the single bed at one or other venue twice a week! In the first four years after qualification they moved around, started a family, worked for higher qualifications and made plans about working in India. There was no time to think about weakness and nothing intruded to cause a re-examination of the changes in life style.

The Indian interlude was associated with a considerable time in bed and a dramatic return to London, but he was unaware of any change in strength until convalescence on the South Coast. He had felt generally weak through the illness and weight loss. He became aware when walking by the sea that he was not walking very fast, and that he could not run. He put this down to general loss of fitness and thought little further about it.

He subsequently became aware of being a little slower, but the dramatic episodes of sudden falls in the street were probably responsible for the self-examination that Sunday morning.

Many years have elapsed since the diagnosis was made. The disease has progressed gradually, and there has been a continuous process of adjustment to increasing weakness. When this increases slowly the natural history of progression is difficult to monitor except in retrospect. The highlights are the development of increasing functional barriers. One remembers what was possible at points in the past compared with what is possible now. Examples are a reduction in walking speed and distance; the ability to mount steps, rise from lying, standing up from a chair and rising from lavatories. Upper limb weakness can be charted by ease of throwing, carrying things, eating, combing one's hair, pulling collars down and unscrewing bottles.

I can walk a few steps with support. I am unable to do more and have become a full time wheelchair user. I use an electric wheelchair. The disabilities that arise from weakness are covered elsewhere, but I refer to them briefly here. In generalised muscle weakness anything that involves the exercise of power will result in major problems in daily living that erode independence.

The overall result is that increasing mental energy is spent assessing whether one can cope with any unfamiliar environment. Chairs are inspected for their shape, height and location in the room. Bathrooms and lavatories must be inspected, and it is no longer possible to get out of a bath even with a special seat and assistance. Access to buildings requires assessment, including churches. The home and office environment are tailored to make life easier. For some years, I had electric office chairs which rose to allow me to stand with less effort, but these are no longer adequate. The strain on ligaments and joints has led to chronic pain.

This pattern is not unusual in the context of neuromuscular disease. The people I have seen as patients confirm my experiences. We all have to take the decision about how much effort we will make to keep going. Sometimes, I catch myself wondering whether it is worth making the effort of will to stand up or do something which will exhaust me. In the early days after the diagnosis had been made I tried physiotherapy, mainly quadriceps strengthening exercises. All this achieved was exhaustion without benefit and I was then unable to concentrate on anything else.

I do not believe religious dualism is an adequate account of humanity; by this, I mean the belief that we contain a separate immaterial entity that we may call spirit or soul. We are physical entities and our spiritual quest emerges from this. I know of no convincing evidence for 'ghosts in machines'. Dualism is not a requirement for a religious outlook on life and the true Judaeo-Christian perspective is non-dualist. Yet, when your body will not do what it is told it is easy to see how people adopt dualism. If the muscles of your body do not work properly on command your body seems divorced from your mind, a useless appendage that is not part of you. Those who sustain acute insults such as stroke, or paralysis due to spinal injury, feel acutely this problem of body image. Those with chronic progressive diseases are in a process of continuous adaptation; they cannot stand still and say they have reintegrated themselves, because the next functional loss will require renewed attempts to keep the body as an integral part of the self.

There is temptation to reject a weak and horrible body, to hate and disown it. There is no easy answer to this; it is a continuing struggle. One can provide some statements based on received religious orthodoxy, but unless they are part of experience, they mean nothing. One can say that God loves the whole of his creation. He loves and suffers with those who are blighted by the risk involved in creating a world like ours. The symbol of Jesus on the cross, rising without his wounds removed, is a powerful reminder that there are no magic answers to suffering in creation. Yet these words are empty if we do not experience the love of others in our lives. I have been angry and bitter, but I have been rescued from that by being loved by my wife and family and having real friends. I have been able to touch and be touched and express myself physically. For much of the time my body, with its impairments and disability, is me. I have ceased to be the young aspiring athlete who loved the physical exultation of exercise and sport. The story of what I have been is part of the narrative of my life that I value and is part of the whole.

Accepting what you are is a continuous process, for we all change. I remember an eighty-year-old man coming to see me in outpatients who had a mild peripheral neuropathy, causing some clumsiness in his hands. "I cannot understand why this should happen to me," he said. He had great difficulty in accepting the change in his body image, the image of himself as a fit and active person.

Integration in the presence of disease is never easy and we move in and out of the ideal. In an acute event the loss of the me or self is sudden. For those with chronic diseases, there is more time to adjust and let go the self that once existed.

Healing relates to making the transition from one old self to the new self. The new self contains the past, but needs to live in the present. Naturally, we all hope that the appropriate treatment will cure us, but there are diseases, many of them affecting the nervous system, where there is no cure.

I refer to healing and cure elsewhere but it is relevant in the context of weakness. Undue emphasis on cure can do serious harm to those seeking to become themselves in a new situation. The Church's healing ministry sometimes seeks to cure where medicine has failed. The theological basis for this seems to be fixed on Jesus' healing miracles. We know little about them and they were performed and interpreted in a cultural setting when miracle workers were common enough. A distorted emphasis on miraculous healing does not help anyone with an incurable disease to experience wholeness, the reverse. This aberrant type of healing ministry results from 'tunnel vision'. It is easy to cite apparent examples of healing miracles and they may well have been miraculous to those concerned. However, God is not a magician and the danger lies in isolating 'miracles' from the overall human experience of disease and suffering.

I have seen people cured and healed in this life, but I have never witnessed a convincing supernatural intervention. I would be puzzled if arbitrary healing did occur. God is in his creation all the time, in good times and bad. He is working with those who seek to make medical advances; he is with us when we emphasise the whole person; he is present when we debate life's priorities, including how we spend our money on research. He is with us in the whole of life. We do not need to separate off a ministry of healing; allowing God into the whole of life is healing.

A real worshipping community will show care for people within and without the community who are in need. The key to healing is acceptance of ourselves, acceptance by others, grounded in our acceptance unconditionally by God.

Healing or integration does not occur always. I recall two completely different people with the same progressive neurological disease, motor neurone disease, causing profound weakness and death within several years. James was a relatively young man in his late thirties, married with a young family. He developed weakness of one leg, but over eighteen months this weakness spread to his whole body, and he became unable to speak or swallow or move his limbs. He was very distressed and his wife, acting as his advocate, was very angry. "How could this happen to anyone?" she asked. She railed against God, me, anyone around. She was desperate for her husband to be cured and he felt the same way. They would latch on to any treatment mentioned. She took her husband to Moscow, where there had been one of the many 'false trails' that occur in the field of incurable diseases. There was no peace; yet their anger was understandable. When bad things happen like this it is normal to be angry and want to blame someone or something. Healing does involve transcending our initial responses.

Simon had spent some time helping to look after a neighbour with terminal multiple sclerosis. Each night, he would help put his friend to bed and he played an important role in caring for him. The neighbour died and not long after Simon developed slurring of his speech, followed by weakness in his limbs. It was apparent that he had motor neurone disease. He continued his work as a surveyor for as long as he could and insisted on taking the collection up at evensong in his parish church until he could hardly walk. He was a man of even temperament and a good sense of humour. Anger was not his style. He had been close to those who suffered, and he had no illusions about the harshness of life. He suffered, but he could know peace.

I have been aware in my work of patients ministering to me and Simon was one of them. He left me feeling humbled and inadequate but better for his coming. He loved life; he did not want to die, but he was never bitter or, at least, I was never aware of it.

Perhaps part of the difference between these two is that one of them did not take life or health for granted. Both are gifts. The one had had an experience of caring and giving himself for another and had seen a dear friend struck down. He did not expect that he had the 'right' to anything different.

It is likely that our temperaments do influence our capacity to cope with adversity, but our acquired attitudes, influenced by the way we live our lives as well as our genetic makeup, have a role in determining how we face disease. How we care for others does influence the way we respond to life events in our own personal world.

Weakness brings with it uncertainty not certainty. The course of the underlying disease itself may be highly unpredictable. Uncertainty became a part of my life at many levels. Muscular dystrophy itself is a very variable disease. I was once informed that I would be a wheelchair user by the time I was forty and would have to retire. The person who told me was one of the world experts on muscle disease. Multiple sclerosis, the cause of a different kind of weakness, is a classic example of an unpredictable neurological disease that makes it very difficult for the person involved to know initially what will happen to them.

There comes a point, particularly in a novel environment, when one can never be sure that one's limbs will carry out the act required. This can cause all sorts of difficulties like getting trapped in 'loos', being unable to control one's bladder for an appropriate length of time, getting stuck in a chair, being unable to access steps one thought one might manage and so on.

A world full of uncertainty can cause one to clutch on to certainties of a religious nature. It may be comforting to hold on to a tightly knit framework when all around one is disintegrating, but that is disconnected from reality and is illusory. For me, this has led to a movement away from religious certainty. I have been compelled to take an open-ended journey towards the mystery of our existence, the source of all being, while remaining within the framework of a specific religion.

Falling

"The Lord upholds all who fall and lifts up all who are bowed down."
Psalm 145.14

"We stumble and fall constantly even when we are most enlightened. But when we are in true spiritual darkness, we do not even know that we have fallen."
Thomas Merton

From the age of 30 he fell repeatedly. In a bad year he would have up to twenty falls. The impact was devastating. He lost complete confidence in his ability to walk safely. In the early years he would fall forwards onto one or other forefoot, forcibly extending his metatarsal joints, resulting in fractures and severe bruising. No one outside the family was aware of the disruption and loss of confidence. He gave up attending the accident and emergency department. In later years he sustained multiple fractures of legs, culminating in a fractured neck of femur that terminated his walking, resulting in full time wheelchair use. These falls spanned forty years and changed his life. It was no longer possible to believe in any kind of certainty.

The Hebrew Bible and the New Testament are replete with rich symbolic use of the word 'fall', 'falling' or 'fallen'. Some quotations may appear positive, others negative. In our language, 'fallen man or woman' and 'upright person' suggest a link between posture and worth. The *Fall* recorded in the book of Genesis is an account of human departure from a perfect state. The impression is that it is possible to be protected from 'falling' if one is righteous, but the fallen state is equated with sin. On the other hand, 'we fall in love'. The common denominator that links references to falling is lack of control; whereas being upright, suggests stability. My falls were a symbol of loss of control.

Everyone falls from time to time, and falling is an essential part of the process of learning to walk. Young children fall and pick themselves up and we thrill at the sight of a new life taking on the adventure of human mobility. The negative side of falling is seen in old age and in people with serious mobility problems; injury is common. One of the most significant injuries of later years is fractured neck of femur due to a simple fall, but with serious implications for future health and mobility. Recurrent falling is not only a physical threat; it endangers the self, impeding the path towards integration and wholeness. The significance of recurrent falling goes beyond the observed event.

Younger people who fall unpredictably, usually have a neurological disorder. Muscular dystrophy is a relatively rare cause of falling in adults, because the disease is uncommon, and in many instances the affected person becomes a wheelchair user before adult life.

People fall for a number of reasons. Ataxia due to disease of the balancing part of the brain called the cerebellum and its pathways may cause falls due to severe unsteadiness of the limbs or trunk. Falls may occur because the foot is weak and the toes scuff the ground. In muscular dystrophy falling is usually due to weakness in the proximal muscles of the lower limbs, notably the hip and quadriceps groups. The usual cause in an ambulant adult with muscular dystrophy is quadriceps weakness. The weakened muscle is unable to cope with undulations underfoot and the leg will suddenly give way at the knee. The reflex is absent and the corrective action is impossible. Because of this and the weak muscles, people 'fall over a sixpence'. It is possible to reduce the number of falls significantly by retaining a high awareness of risk and watching the ground all the time. This requires intense mental concentration.

Karen was in her mid-twenties when I first saw her. She had a young son, but a problematic marriage. Karen's mother had a neuromuscular disease, but it was mild and had had no major impact on daily life. Karen's problems were worse. She was prone to sudden falls in awkward places. She had fallen crossing the road and in shops. The falls were due to very weak quadriceps muscles that destabilised her knees. Her hip flexors were weak also. Karen found these falls very distressing. She would get angry and noted that no one seemed particularly interested. "I expect people think I have had one too many", she would say. Her weight was not excessive. There was no specific treatment other than to advise her to think about every step she took, consider the possibility of using a stick and examining her footwear. Karen became depressed and required medication.

George had a different disease. A rare disorder of balance termed Friedrich's Ataxia. George was fourteen when we first met. Even then he walked with a very unsteady gait. It was quite alarming to see him as he staggered around, giving the impression that he would fall at any time. George was very independent, resourceful and intelligent. He did well academically and was offered a place to study a scientific subject at a local university. By then he had passed a driving test and drove an automatic car.

His walking deteriorated. Friedrich's Ataxia is a complex disorder and may have other features, including weakness. George was falling more often. He fractured his ankle. He was determined to go to university, but when he visited he was aware of access problems into the scientific block. The distance between buildings was greater than his walking allowed. He accepted for the first time that he could not be safe without becoming a partial wheelchair user. However, it still proved difficult for him to continue with his course, and after some months he found it impossible to cope with the stress.

Sudden repetitive falls have the potential to create post-traumatic stress that never settles entirely because of the occurrence of the next episode. The worst part of this is the flashes that intrude into the mind at unexpected moments when one relives the injuries.

I have discussed falling with people who have come to see me. Their experience is very similar. Apart from the pain, the first reaction is of humiliation and anger. Most people want to be left alone for a short while, partly to assess any injuries and to compose themselves. When weakness is well established, it is impossible to rise from the ground independently. In the earlier stages of muscular dystrophy, it is possible to 'climb up oneself', but otherwise there needs to be someone who can heave one onto a chair or push one in the behind as one makes the effort to get up. When I have fallen with no one around, I have sometimes had to roll into a ball until I could get myself nearer to some physical help; an example was rolling towards and partly down a river bank until I could gain enough mechanical advantage to stand up.

The anger is difficult to analyse. In part, it is due to loss of dignity and frustration that something has happened despite expending great energy trying to avoid it. The anger is 'free floating', not intentionally directed, although the hapless person in the way bears the brunt.

I do not feel particularly ashamed of being angry, although I am ashamed of being angry with loved ones. There is no point in directing the anger towards God; He is not there, or is He? In a way the loved one serves as a proxy figure against whom one can rail. All that anyone can do is to stand by while the adjustment takes place again. The role of friend and family is supportive in this way. There is no solution to falling except ceasing to walk; loved ones cannot cure progressive diseases and neither can God, but awareness of support enables acceptance.

I find that the only way I can live with all this and retain a belief in the presence of God is to accept the limitations imposed on him by his own nature, and that he does not intervene in our world. The uncertainty created by falls does have an impact on simplistic attributes that are so readily applied to God or our gods. The one characteristic that we all hang on to is the idea of a loving God. What is the basis for knowing what loving can really mean in this context? One traditional response is that in Jesus we see the human face of God. The life of Jesus suggests he was concerned about others and particularly those in need. His teaching suggests a reordering of society where the disadvantaged are no longer oppressed. However, the remoteness of Jesus as a historical figure makes it difficult to know any detail about his life. We are left to dwell on the actions and attitudes of people in our world if we are to approach any understanding of what love might mean

In life, we all have experiences, if we are fortunate, of compassion, selflessness, giving, steadfastness, self-sacrifice and other attributes we might want to apply to the highest forms of love. These qualities exist. We would assume that someone with these gifts, that seem to be found in Jesus, would have a strong desire to take away the suffering of others. Every time a member of our family suffers we long to take away their pain and even bear it ourselves. Yet this kind of love is impotent to change the bad things in life. That love cannot remove disease. We have to realise also that every quality that we describe is a human quality. There is no possibility of being sure that the word 'love', as applied to the ultimate Godhead, is anything like the love we conceive on earth. We long to use this word love, but perhaps we should use it less. I have concluded that if we are able to experience God, attributes no longer have the same importance.

Falling is a challenge to certainty and integration. The occasional fall is unlikely to become a major issue, but repeated falls pose the question: How one can maintain the self in the face of this lack of control? We function by having a reasonable working knowledge of how to cope with the physical environment and the limitations of our bodies. Above a certain level of unpredictability, the degree of uncertainty created is destructive. For example, if one is unsure whether the body will function safely in a setting, the obvious way out is to retreat from the situation. In the context of ambulation this means adopting a means of transport which may meet the environmental challenge. The alternative is to restrict the environment and never travel alone. An analysis of my own falls has questioned any simple strategy. They are unpredictable and I have fallen as much within the home as outside.

I use falling as a symbol of uncertainty and risk. I do not readily connect with any biblical imagery about falling and uprightness. Much of the time, when I am deciding whether to do something or not, I feel as if I am on a piece of elastic. Interest and initial motivation may encourage me to explore a possible avenue, and then the recoil starts. This happens when I consider the physical risk, the uncertainty of the environment, and my ability to cope with the unknown.

Reflecting on the whole business, I realise that frailty enables us to think about the fragility of human existence. For much of the time we immure ourselves from the reality that we are vulnerable and personal control of our lives can be broken in a moment.

Humility is a very difficult word. It certainly does not mean a cringing, self-apologetic attitude. It does seem to involve a realistic acceptance of the sort of people we are, our true position in the universe as finite creatures; our dependence on living in community, and a clear acceptance of our capacity to make mistakes.

Status and worldly success can lure us into the illusion of invulnerability; give us the impression we can sort anything out. Falling symbolises our fragile hold on the world, but like many other unpleasant experiences we can learn positive things.

Disability and Healing

"Your wound is incurable, your injury beyond healing.
There is no one to plead your cause, no remedy for your sore,
no healing for you."
Jeremiah 30.13

"Jesus went through all the towns and villages, teaching in their
synagogues, preaching the good news of the kingdom and
healing every disease and illness."
Matthew 9.35

These quotations expose much of the confusion that lies at the
heart of debate about healing through religion. Some people need
to believe that there is someone in control out there who will cure
all ailments if they follow the right formulae.

The reference in Jeremiah may well refer to the spiritual
state of the nation of Judah, but it takes a harsher view of God
than is suggested by the works of Jesus, recorded in Matthew's
Gospel. Jeremiah exposes the links between conduct and healing
that exist in the minds of many, but not born out by the
experience of the man Job in the Hebrew Bible. In the biblical
account of his trials there is never any real doubt that Job was a
good person, although his friends' need to maintain theological
orthodoxy caused them to insist that he must have sinned in some
way.

One can understand how some people reading the New Testament of the Bible, and taking it at 'face value', believe that all diseases can be healed whatever medical opinion holds.

The difficulty with this viewpoint is that it runs counter to the experience of the many millions of people who encounter or experience for themselves incurable disease. It is not possible for me and many like me to ignore the reality of severe disability and explain it away as being due to sin, lack of faith, God's will or any other set of platitudes.

Any book like this one is bound to have references to healing, but I have chosen to focus some comments on healing in the context of disability. This is because the word 'disability' has very wide-ranging implications for any serious consideration of healing and 'wholeness' as opposed to cure.

Disability is essentially related to how we function in daily living and in society. It is not a word that is disease specific. The word disability is used to indicate functional difficulties that arise through mental and physical disease. It is intended to mean something connected with abnormality. The phrase 'we are all disabled' may appear meaningful, but it distracts from the reality that some people have difficulties that lie well outside normal experience.

If one considers the world-wide impact of disability there is no doubt about the huge problem that exists. In a developed country the main impact of disability is amongst elderly people. In developing countries, poverty, malnutrition and serious infection cause disability in children and younger people. War has had a major impact on disability both in military and civilian populations.

In medicine, the whole subject of disability should be dictated by functional considerations. When I was younger, the traditional model of neurological practice was based on a detailed history and examination. Once a diagnosis had been made the whole question of treatment remained problematical. Many conditions remained incurable and rehabilitation and disease management were poorly developed. Neurology had the reputation of an esoteric subject providing considerable intellectual satisfaction, but offering little practical help to the victims of the fascinating disorders under study.

Although diagnostic neurology remains important, it is now accepted that function is an overriding issue once the diagnosis has been made. All forms of intervention must be evaluated on whether they improve function in a measurable way, or improve quality of life by reducing distressing symptoms. Although disease identification is important because specific treatment may be indicated, the emphasis of long term rehabilitation and care is functional and multidisciplinary. At any one time one discipline may be more important than another. In some situations the medical model of care is undesirable. In general, the further removed the subject is from an acute event the less need for medical involvement there is. This is not the case in progressive diseases that require continued assessment or monitoring of long term medication. As treatments for previously untreatable diseases become available more medical intervention will be required. Neurology is a dynamic changing subject, increasingly concerned with improving the disabilities of those with severe neurological disorders.

The words disability, impairment and handicap have reasonably specific meanings. Politically correct use of words has become an issue. The phrase 'mental handicap' is not acceptable, but the phrase a person with 'learning difficulties' is, because it describes the problem that someone has and not their social disadvantage.

Words such as 'epileptic', 'the disabled' and 'the handicapped' do not appeal to people who live in these situations. One might ask why it matters so much when the intentions are right? We can certainly become over obsessed with political correctness in language, but the reason for the sensitivity lies in a long history of paternalism towards people with disabilities. There is a failure also to recognise that everyone who has a difficulty has their own individual set of impairments, disabilities and handicaps. It may appear pedantic to say someone has epilepsy rather than saying that he is an epileptic, but the word 'epileptic' hides a whole world of prejudice and discrimination which has discredited it.

Attitudes to disease and disability are steeped in historical prejudice in which religious and cultural factors have been very important. Disease has commonly been identified as punishment for sin. One explanation for bad things happening to people is that disease and disability represent divine retribution. Mental illness has been identified with moral depravity or demon possession. Epilepsy has been regarded in the same way. The clinical presentation of someone in a generalised convulsion has been linked with spirit possession.

Prosperity and good health have been linked with good behaviour. It is difficult to overestimate the social disadvantage of disability, even in the modern world.

The word impairment describes the specific weakness or area of abnormality: paralysis of the arm is impairment.

Disability results from this. Someone with a paralysed arm may be having difficulty in lifting objects, carrying, dressing and manipulating articles. Handicap describes the major disadvantage of living in an environment where it is not possible to alleviate the disability because of inaccessibility, lack of resources or social barriers.

The first person who made an impact on me through disability was Albert. At our teaching hospital, which was not large, he was an important figure in the life of a young intern. Albert had been a student and just after qualification had developed severe paralytic poliomyelitis. He was left with profound impairments and disabilities. He was a continuous wheelchair user. He was unable to breathe adequately without using a respirator at night. He had marked upper limb weakness.

Albert lived in the hospital. He had a role running the anticoagulant clinics and helped on particular wards. He was a very kind man. He always had a word of advice and support. I never knew him well, but he made a deep impression on me. He was around a good deal during my first job. I suppose I was afraid to talk to him personally. He wore a beard, but one detected the signs of weariness and depression on his face. Perhaps we were all too preoccupied with ourselves to come near him. Everything became too much for him eventually and he decided to die.

Whatever the collective failures in communicating with and supporting Albert, the hospital had found him a role and made him part of that living community. Despite his very severe impairments and disabilities he was retained as a valued member of the hospital and this reduced his handicap. All that seems rather old fashioned now. Today be might be retired on medical grounds; told he was unfit to do anything safely. Whatever legislation we may pass, it is still necessary to be positive about a person's potential; to make inroads into the world of discrimination.

One of the issues surrounding disability is this question: How severe does it have to be before someone is unable to function at all in this world? Events take over. Passivity is all that can be displayed. It may be argued that few people are that disabled. But someone in a 'vegetative state' can do nothing for himself or herself. At this point one is dependent on the attitudes and actions of others, either to remain alive, or die.

I suppose it depends on how one reads the Gospels, but one hallmark of the ministry of Jesus was sympathy and understanding of the poor and disadvantaged. Most of us read the Bible in a very selective way, but if we are to make anything of a social gospel the Bible is supportive. Although, as far as we know, Jesus did not have a physical or mental impairment of note, he did one thing that resonates with those who are unable to help themselves. After his ordeal in the Garden of Gethsemane he gave himself up to the authorities, or rather it is recorded that he was betrayed. The account of Jesus' trial and crucifixion may be read as amounting to a surprising level of passivity on his part. Although the way the story is dramatized may suggest this, I prefer to understand the account as an example of how people become dependent on the attitude and behaviour of others in determining the outcome. I have never been attracted to a picture of Jesus consciously walking to a pre-determined destiny, acting the part that was written for him. I can empathise with him being true to his message, and unwilling to compromise the spiritual truths he preached. Threats to his life did not deter him. There came a point when he allowed his life and work to speak for itself. He was arrested, and the conduct of those that arrested and tried him, together with the attitude of a faction of the local populace, determined his outcome. This surrender has some contact with the position of those who have to give their lives up and trust in the goodness of others. There comes a point for all of us when we can do no more for our cause, or for ourselves. In the end life and death, or justice, are not dependent on the individual, but the role of the community.

The picture of Sarah, her family and the Pope is still on my desk. Her parents gave it to me after she died. We had managed to keep her going long enough to make her journey by ambulance to Rome to see and be blessed by the Pope. She died soon after returning home. She was twenty-five. Multiple sclerosis had killed her.

I first met her when she was sixteen and studying for her A levels. She had had an episode of double vision and this had slowly started to improve. Even at this early stage of the disease clinical examination revealed more widespread neurological signs than were suggested by the symptoms. Investigation indicated a diagnosis of multiple sclerosis.

Unfortunately, the disease progressed rapidly. Courses of steroid drugs were ineffective. Sarah became very unsteady and her legs were stiff and weak. She developed a severe tremor of her arms. She was unable to pass urine normally. Within two years of her first symptoms she was a wheelchair user.

The disease soon affected mental function. Memory became severely impaired. Sarah remained cheerful and smiling. Her mood was inappropriate. The medical term for this is euphoria. Many people with multiple sclerosis are depressed, but some that have very severe disease are euphoric.

Sarah was unable to do anything for herself and this included thinking. Her family provided total support. She was steeped in the traditions of the Roman Catholic Church. The liturgy and practice of the Church were the truths that she had lived by, along with her family. The faith and love of her local worshipping community sustained her. The experience of her illness was lived out through collective awareness of the presence of God. I never encountered bitterness or anger from any member of the family. Sarah was forced to give herself up to love and care. Was this healing?

The pattern of a slowly progressive muscle disease became clearer in retrospect. Until he was thirty his disabilities had a minor impact on daily living. A sedentary existence masked problems other than his ability to play games.

The gradual evolution of disability and handicap began to impact on him thereafter. Although his face, arms, trunk and legs were involved, the dramatic falls were the events with the most impact on his life.

He would fall in the street, in restaurants, the house and garden. He was unable to get up and required physical assistance. The inevitable injuries occurred. A succession of fractures eroded independence, creating handicap. Eventually he abandoned much of his independent travel. He became unable to walk down the street alone. He started to use a stick and then crutches. He managed to stay on his feet until his late sixties, but serious lower limb fractures necessitated wheelchair use. The wheelchair facility included a seat riser that allowed standing.

The disabilities arising from upper limb weakness had a major impact on daily living. He could not eat tidily with a knife and fork and frequently used a spoon. The inability to elevate his arms above the horizontal meant that he could not lift a heavy cup, had problems doing up buttons and turning down collars. When he took church services his wife or other helpers had to put on his robes. When he became a wheelchair user he required help manipulating communion vessels at certain times. In the home environment, he was unable to carry plates or drinks, open bottles, unscrew caps. His wife had to lead in any social encounter involving hospitality.

The general consequences of his impairments affected many other aspects of daily life.

Bathroom facilities had to be modified. He could not get out of a bath even with a bath aid. A wheelchair/ walk in shower was installed. A 'normal' lavatory was inadequate. He required a speciality 'loo' with an electric seat rise that enabled him to stand and reach his wheelchair

He became unable to get out of an ordinary car. Initially he was able to use a large 4x4 vehicle. Eventually this became impossible and a wheelchair accessible vehicle was used with a hoist for the chair, and a sophisticated vehicle seat that rotated out of the vehicle. His wife had to load the chair.

He discovered that there were major issues accessing other peoples' homes, even those of his children, with an electric chair. This resulted in an increasing amount of social isolation. He was a 'loner' by nature, but even so it depressed him

He had enjoyed travel by air to exotic destinations, but airports and the planes themselves became a major challenge. There was extreme difficulty getting out of a plane seat. On a number of occasions he became stranded and was dependent on ground staff to assist him. The lack of upper limb strength meant *that his handicap was different to someone with a paraplegia and normal upper limbs.*

Overall, he began to empathise with those who wanted to withdraw from life. The stress associated with social activity readily caused anxiety and agitation.

Anyone with a disability that disadvantages them in life will reflect on the unfairness of it all; the random nature of so much that happens to them, unless they take a world view that understands all events to be in the purpose and will of God. There are no rational explanations as to why 'bad things happen to good people.'

In some circumstances it is possible to identify happenings attributable to human behaviour, but this is not the case in many human diseases. They are part of the fabric of creation at the time we live in the creative process. The resultant disability happens in a world where most of the people do not have disabilities, and the structure of society is ordered for the majority. However, increasing longevity is resulting in many frailer people, and technical developments have resulted in a new generation of children and young adults damaged by disease and accidents. At our present state of knowledge there seems little evidence that disability is on the wane.

Impairment and disability can frighten unaffected people who are unfamiliar with such difficulties. Barriers to real communication develop; people who have disabilities can become angry at the way they are treated. A friend of mine disabled by severe multiple sclerosis used to become angry at the banal but well-meaning remarks offered to her by an archdeacon who visited her. "You are so brave my dear", was the kind of remark that enraged her. She felt she was not being treated like an ordinary person. Her illness had erected a barrier between her and the venerable cleric that reflected his inadequacy in the presence of disease and disability. She was left to help him conduct himself in a more relaxed manner.

Much time and effort is expended finding solutions to problems. This is hard graft. The whole point about chronic disability is that the disease process is not treatable. The cause may be a one-off event such as traumatic brain injury or a chronic disease such as multiple sclerosis, Parkinson's disease or dementia. The people involved have no prospect of cure in the current state of knowledge, and if they are to make connections with the Christian gospel, the emphasis must be on wholeness in their present situation and the progressive deterioration that may lie ahead. Undue emphasis on interventionist models of the healing ministry has nothing to offer those who are not going to get better. A patient of mine with multiple sclerosis became involved with a Christian group who wanted to cure her with the laying on of hands. The result was disillusionment and anger. The son of a lifelong friend abandoned his medical follow up for a spinal cord tumour and was taken to an American evangelist; he was a 'healer'; nothing happened. Treatment was delayed and may have resulted in increased disability.

It is not possible to know what happened in the Gospel healing miracles; their relevance to the issue of how God works in the world should never be separated from ordinary experience and other aspects of the Gospels. Jesus did not rescue himself and his experience during the story of his temptations would seem to cast serious doubt on the interpretation of the miraculous in the Gospel stories. The Devil was not permitted to rescue Jesus from his hunger, or provide easy worldly power and magical answers to predicaments.

Providence is the word technically used for the action of God in the world. In a busy life involving thousands of patients I remember Sarah, particularly in the context of divine intervention. For me, she became a symbol of the silence of God. God does not intervene supernaturally in this world. Maurice Wiles, in his Bampton lectures, wrote instructively on the issue of Providence. It makes little sense to imagine the intervention of God in some lives and not in others. If God is present throughout creation, he is there always. He does not interfere some of the time. True spirituality can never depend on an intervening god in one's own life. We are all too aware of the massive natural tragedies to make any sense at all of a god who intervenes sometimes and not others. We may conclude, either that we are in the presence of a deep mystery that keeps our search for the Divine alive, or abandon the project.

People with severe disability have the possibility of greater wholeness, but it depends on others whether much of this happens. Practical improvements in accessibility, employment attitudes and a general understanding of potential would help. If humans are to transcend the status of the rest of the animal world they need to accept the weak as part of them rather than a separate part of creation.

In Vincent Donavon's book *Rediscovering Christianity,* there is a picture of the Masai village community and their attitude to baptism. The priest is taken to task for dwelling on individual worth; the strength and weaknesses of the community are brought together in a collective decision, either everyone will be baptised or no one.

The core of a genuine Christian outlook is the realisation that our own wellbeing, salvation, healing, cannot exist if we are unaware and uncaring of the needs of others. A primary Christian goal is concerned with inclusiveness not exclusiveness. True wholeness is about completing the circle, with all included as points on it.

Sex and Disability

"Of all the sexual aberrations, chastity is the strangest."
Anatole France

It may seem too obvious to remind anyone that all human beings are sexual beings regardless of the level and type of their disability. It is necessary because there is a long social and medical history of ignoring and even discouraging such a notion. People with disabilities may be regarded as unable to have sexual intercourse through physical or mental limitation. They may receive no support or encouragement in experiencing their own sexuality. Young people with disabilities are often cut off from the usual adolescent explorations of their sexual nature. For many people the thought of passionate sexual activity between severely disabled people is repulsive, not to be discussed. Disabled people may even be regarded as having abnormal sexual cravings. A common misapprehension is that people with disabilities inevitably produce a disabled child.

Sadly, neither the clergy or health care professionals have a good record in helping people with disabilities find sexual fulfilment.

John had multiple sclerosis. Although he could still walk a few yards, drive a car and work in his job as director of a small business, he was distressed by impotence. He was married with a young family. His wife was very supportive. Unlike many people he did not find it difficult to talk about his sexual difficulties. He was unable to sustain an erection. In addition, he had significant bladder symptoms although he was continent for much of the time and could empty his bladder.

He found his inability to have successful sexual intercourse with his wife a major loss. He wished to explore all possible avenues of assistance. His libido was normal and his sexual difficulties were due to neurological damage to the spinal cord.

At around this time work had just commenced on a trial of injecting papaverine, a vasodilator drug, into the corpus cavernosum of the penis. It was shown that providing the dose was titrated for each person, it was possible to obtain an erection for sufficient time to allow successful intercourse. The main problem was the possibility of a prolonged and painful erection; this would require drainage of blood from the dorsal vein of the penis to relieve the problem. Despite the inconvenience of the procedure and one or two mishaps with prolonged erections, John found the treatment very helpful and his quality of life much improved. He subsequently moved on to using less direct means through medication.

That example of sexual problems in relation to disabling neurological disease is relatively simple. The subject was married already and in a conventional family situation. Many people with neurological disease are deprived of sexual expression for much more difficult reasons. Early life disease and disability may leave people physically and mentally impaired. There may be a strong desire for sexual experience. However, social reality limits opportunities for relationships.

Alice had epilepsy and mild neurological impairments without undermining her independence. Despite extensive specialist interventions her seizures were not fully controlled. She had a mixture of major attacks and complex partial seizures in which she would lose awareness and carry out automatic motor acts. Alice took regular anticonvulsant medication. She had been unable to obtain employment despite having secretarial skills. She had her own flat, supportive parents and received various disability benefits.

Alice found social contact and friendships very difficult to establish. This concerned her greatly. She was very brave about it, but desperately lonely. Attempts were made to facilitate contacts through various clubs and social outlets. She tried going to church, but this did not help her with friendships.

Eventually, through a club she met Paul. He had epilepsy as well. He had greater physical disability than Alice and he was less able generally. They became friends and then lovers and moved into a council flat together. Alice was very supportive and protective of Paul. There was no doubt that this relationship meant a lot to Alice. She was much happier and her seizure frequency reduced dramatically. She required less medication.

A cynic might argue that such relationships are fragile; that they are doomed to fail in the long term; that it would be irresponsible for such people to have children. I can see no real reason for denying Alice and Paul a loving relationship that has helped them transcend their loneliness. Although one would wish such friendships to last, it may be unwise to insist that longevity is the only mark of quality in human friendship. Alice and Paul have experienced sexual and emotional fulfilment that cannot be taken away.

In his book *Embodiment,* James B Nelson quotes a number of accounts about the importance of sexuality in terminal states or severe disability. He agrees with Louis Jaffe, a professor of social work, who considers that it is quite erroneous that terminal illness precludes sexual desire. This may continue to be present. Paradoxically, libido may increase during or after a severe illness. However, this may remain unrecognised or ignored by professional carers and family.

Loss or difficulty in expressing one's sexuality is a form of death. The physical expression of sexual being is life enhancing, stress reducing and part of being human.

Imagine a young person male or female who has a severe neurological disorder, for example cerebral palsy. As that young person matures physically and emotionally he or she enters adolescence in the same way as anyone else. But for many there are great problems in fulfilling their desires and longings. Social isolation is commonplace. Their sexuality is forgotten by others or not discussed. There is a vague hope that they may find someone disabled like themselves and form worthwhile friendships and sexual relationships. Sometimes, whatever happens, there is doubt about conventional marriage being the ideal solution in many situations. Very severe disability may make this unrealistic. Why not allow young people with severe disabilities to enjoy sex without judging the legal status of their relationship?

Orthodox Christianity regards sexual fidelity and marriage as the norm. Extramarital sex, despite current cultural practice, is generally not spoken about freely by clergy. One can certainly argue that an ideal is monogamous marriage for life, but there are many reasons why this ideal is unrealised. Amongst able-bodied people there are those who find it very difficult to remain with one partner only. Some people have a level of sexual drive that makes it very difficult for them to remain monogamous. This is not intended to undermine the Christian ideal of marriage, but in the context of those with profound disability it is vital to ask questions. What good can be realised through relationships or sexual expression that do not meet this ideal? Is it appropriate for any religion to impose an ordinance of abstention from sexual activity if these ideals cannot realistically be met?

The various levels of sexual contact involve increasing physical intimacy. Physical contact is extremely important for anyone with a physical disability. The person with a profound level of impairment, most often neurological, is likely to have a low level of self-esteem, to be afraid that their appearance is repugnant to others and that their functional limitations are unlikely to make them attractive to anyone. This is a real issue, but there are people who are able to transcend these barriers and see beyond the conventional models of beauty and attractiveness. It is more likely that mutual need will bring people with comparable disabilities together, but one should never discount the possibility of an able-bodied person finding real fulfilment with someone who has a profound physical disability, but it is rare.

This leads to the possibility that physical contact for some people will be at a different level or not at all. Consider the situation of a young person with very severe cerebral palsy; he/she is unable to express himself/herself fully sexually but longs to do so. there is no impairment of mental function and full insight into the predicament. He/she is tired of people saying how wonderful they are and how patient in the face of adversity. What is wanted is to feel and explore a man or woman's body and know that person is happy to be with them. For example, a young man meets a young woman who is very kind and caring. He likes her very much indeed, but he is not in any position to make physical advances and anyway he is quite sure she would be embarrassed and even frightened. She would not know what to do.

One day he hears about a young woman who is a sex therapist. She has become aware of the sexual problems of disabled people. She had a brother who died at a young age of a progressive neurological disease. She is prepared to help people with physical disabilities experience sexual contact. She can help them with their own limitations. It is arranged that she visits him. He finds her very attractive. She tells him that she gets real fulfilment from helping people like him. She can touch him and explore his body without feeling repulsed. They can have sexual intercourse. The experience for him is incredible. She is an angel. He has had an experience that he felt would never fall to him. He loves her for what she has shown to him. She respects him. There is no suggestion of a long-term relationship. There is no commitment to regular sexual activity. He does not care. She has helped him to a special level of experience. He sees God in her.

The Bible does not provide a coherent account of sexual ethics. Those who wish to argue a very conservative stance on human sexuality are able to pick texts that appear to sustain their position, but they omit the ambiguity that exists in the Bible. Old Testament Bible quotations about disability and sexuality have no traction on how we should view these issues in our world. Much of the material contained in Exodus and Leviticus is concerned with the keeping of purity laws and the preservation of the nation. There are practical regulations or taboos about sexual behaviour, but these are mainly concerned with the preservation of the wider family unit. There is no insistence on monogamy. The attitude to sex appears to be practical and realistic apart from the general and sexual prohibitions recorded.

Jesus said very little at all about sexual relations. Paul appears to forbid certain homosexual acts but there is no detailed sexual conduct law that could last for all time. Jesus wanted all relationships to be loving and self-giving, but he does not comment on disability.

A balanced account of the Bible and sexual ethics is provided in *Dirt Greed and Sex* by L William Countryman. He argues that New Testament sexual ethics remained framed in purity and property systems. The context is alien to today's world. Although it may be tempting to use this framework for regulating sexual conduct in the twenty-first century it is basically an abrogation of responsible thought.

As he points out, Jesus was not a systematic teacher. The whole idea that a coherent structure can be derived from Jesus' life and teaching is highly questionable. Jesus was concerned about transforming lives. If we consider the general issue of disability, the Bible has some harsh things to say on the subject. It is appropriate to quote from texts about physical defects as the negative approach would impact on all aspects of life. Levitical law prohibited anyone with a disability drawing near to God:

"For the generations to come none of your descendants who has a defect may come near to offer the food of his God. No man who has any defect may come near: no man who is blind or lame, disfigured or deformed; no man with a crippled foot or hand, or who is a hunchback or a dwarf, or who has any eye defect, or who has festering or running sores or damaged testicles. No descendant of Aaron the priest who has any defect is to come near to present the food offerings to the Lord. He has a defect; he must not come near to offer the food of his God."

Leviticus 21.17-21

It is easy enough to scoff that this ancient law is irrelevant today. But similar attitudes to disability and normal living remain. I recall a distinguished neurology colleague who informed me that someone with epilepsy could never be a priest. He was a Roman Catholic. If it is possible for people to believe that a person with disabilities cannot be a priest, it is easy to suggest that they have diminished rights in other areas including human sexuality. Fortunately, for every bad passage in the Bible there is usually a better one; a significant message for those who insist on quoting texts to justify their beliefs.

"I will make the lame my remnant, those driven away a strong nation. The Lord will rule over them in Mount Zion from that day and for ever."

Micah 4.7

A person of liberal dispositions would not consider homosexuality to be a disability but some people do. Attitudes to gay relationships and sex are very different in the West compared to conservative and traditional cultures in continents such as Africa. The following remarks are based on the prevailing situation in Europe.

The spectrum of sexual orientation is broad; it is self-evident that many of those who are mainly same sex orientated do not consciously choose it. There is a tendency to reduce the complexities of homosexuality to categories. Some people regard it as a disease with the possibility of genetic factors determining it; This raises interesting issues concerning treatment. I regard this approach as inappropriate nowadays. Society is now taking a more enlightened approach to sexual difference and gender identity. At the time I qualified in medicine, there was a vogue for 'treating' male homosexuality with abreaction therapy. The 'patient' would be shown photographs of women or men and punished for the wrong response.

Homosexuality may still be seen as a sin. The word sin can be applied to the latent state of being attracted to the same sex or the sexual act itself. In the Church nowadays there appears to be some acceptance that sexual orientation towards the same sex amongst clergy can be accepted, providing the person remains celibate. Long standing sexual relationships are not encouraged by those of a conservative disposition. This is a gross insult to loving couples. The failure to prefer outstanding priests to episcopal level is deeply disturbing. The refusal to marry same sex couples in the Church of England is equally distressing. The more liberal American Episcopal Church has ignored these restrictions and is producing a common marriage service for heterosexual and homosexual couples. It is very difficult to reconcile restrictive regulations with reality.

The texts in the Bible that comment on same sex relationships are not part of a text book for today. The words of Leviticus relate to purity and property laws from a Hebrew culture. If they are given absolute status regardless of our current knowledge base no form of argument will counter them. But this kind of external authority is in grave danger of being used selectively.

"If a man has sexual relations with a man as one does with a woman, both of them have done what is detestable. They are to be put to death; their blood will be on their own heads."

Leviticus 20.13

There is no obvious reason why sexual ethics should be regarded differently to other ethical issues. The cultural context of the Bible does not exclude slavery but we do not condone it nowadays. There is no overarching framework in scripture to provide answers to today's moral questions. The ethics of Jesus are more concerned with living under the law of love rather than being bound by regulations. Love of God, love of neighbour and a life of concern for others are the hallmarks of a truly Christian morality.

Depression

"Darkling I listen; and for many a time
I have been half in love with easeful Death,
Call'd him soft names in many a mused rhyme,
To take into the air my quiet breath;
Now more than ever seems it rich to die
To cease upon the midnight with no pain,
While thou art pouring forth thy soul abroad
In such ecstacy!
Still woulds't thou sing and I have ears in vain
To thy high requiem become a sod."
John Keats *Ode to A Nightingale*

Disorders of mood are difficult to define and depression means different things to different people. There is more to depression than feeling fed up or having an off day. The natural process of grieving is not depression unless it merges with a depressive disorder after a long time. Depression can mean an absence of feeling, like being in a black hole; it may be numbness, a feeling of being cut off from the world and one's usual self. Sometimes the description of feeling like a machine running on one cylinder describes some aspects of the disease. Agitation, poor sleep and appetite, loss of libido, irritability and weepiness may occur. The onset may be triggered by a life event or the depression comes for no reason. In severe instances the perceived agony and meaninglessness of existence drives the subject to contemplate death as a release from torture.

There is evidence that physical health problems are associated with depression, particularly in susceptible individuals. Because depression is a disease affecting people with unique lives the manifestations vary considerably. Depression and the opposite, mania, are due to a disorder of brain chemistry. The precise mechanism is ill understood, but mood disorders may respond to specific drug therapy.

The young doctor was about twenty-five years old when he had his initial episode of depression. He never realised this at the time. He had been aware of considerable fluctuations of energy and drive previously; periods of intense activity and productivity and others of relative apathy. It lasted for more than a year and then lifted.

There was one child at the time and there was much to be happy about. There had been an acute urinary infection before the depression started and work at the Heart Hospital in London was demanding and stressful. The infection resolved and what was noticeable afterwards was an inability to get going again.

It was easy to blame the recent acute illness, but all the tests were normal. He lost interest in work and sex and wanted to avoid both; sleep pattern altered and usual energy disappeared. As is often the case he interpreted this event in retrospect.

It was a number of years before a more serious and prolonged bout occurred. Even in retrospect it is difficult to determine, what if any, precipitating factors were relevant. He was involved in a very busy job; his mother had died and it was around this time that he had a diagnosis of muscular dystrophy confirmed. The recall of the temporal relevance of these matters is not good.

The main memory was feeling terrible. He was very irritable and feeling extremely low about everything. At the time, he was a deacon at a local Baptist church but ceased to go regularly. He found it difficult to face people although he continued work like an automaton.

One Sunday morning he went to the hospital and straight to his room. He sat in a chair. On his desk were bottles of antidepressant tablets from pharmaceutical representatives. He took them all and then sat and waited. He remembered nothing else until someone started to put a tube down his throat as a prelude to 'washing him out'. The ward sister had happened to come up to the upper storey of the department to tidy his room. The door had no lock and so she found him. She took a major decision to try and keep the matter quiet and had summoned someone from the accident and emergency department to treat him in his room.

She took him home to her house and then told his wife. It was a difficult time. There were four small children and a lot of responsibilities. A psychiatrist friend lived in the same road and he commenced treatment in the doctor's house. Somehow, he kept going to work but the high doses of antidepressants affected speech and blood pressure.

Despite a lot of treatment and support the depression was always there and one further overdose was taken which required resuscitation. The cycle of depression lasted for over two years, but gradually his mood started to lift. The medication was reduced and life became brighter.

Subsequent episodes have occurred. Each attack lasted for about two years. Important features were significant agitation and a feeling of being unable to cope. Irritability was marked. Sleep was severely disturbed. Thinking became more obsessive and ruminative. There was a total absence of calm. He became unable to open the post without agitation.

Every minor problem appeared insoluble and was grossly magnified. Although he recognised that he was depressed it was very difficult for him to be persuaded of his altered view of life until he was better. Each time he recovered he would tell himself that he would be able to recognise that what he thought when he was depressed was not a true picture of the world.

On recovery he would be aware of a blissful calm. Sleep returned to a more normal pattern. He realised that his powers of concentration had been impaired. He felt guilty about the whole thing but it was him. These bouts seemed a kind of curse.

It is very difficult to give an account of depression but it changes life dramatically. One is convinced that the 'depressed' view of the world is the real one. It seems quite reasonable to ask the question, which view of the world is closer to reality? Is there a world view that is anything other than entirely subjective; one that depends on your brain chemicals? It is very disturbing to realise that chemical changes in the brain can alter our picture of ourselves and all around us.

Despite the view, held by some, that mental illness is a 'myth', the mainstream view is that serious mental illness is on a par with physical disease, but this is less obvious because of the complex nature of the brain and cultural and educational factors that influence human behaviour. The manifestations of disease are different because the site of the problem is our brain and thus our whole being is affected. Effective treatment may result in recovery and a recognition that a terrible ordeal is over; the thoughts and feelings experienced were distorted by disease and it is possible to rejoice at the renewal of life.

In his episode of depression in the 1970s institutional religion seemed pointless to the young doctor. He was unable to go and meet people in a worshipping community and he felt he received no real help from the church. The support base was from family and close colleagues

He found the wordy content of any service he attended particularly difficult to cope with; religious language seemed a foreign language with no point of contact that he could recognise. He had an overwhelming feeling of wanting to be quiet and yet the clamour of life seemed to make this impossible. One day, when he was at home and on his own, he had an overwhelming sense of the presence of God. He could not describe it. It was very reassuring. His interpretation of this experience was similar to that recorded in the book of Job.

"I know that you can do all things;
no purpose of yours can be thwarted. You asked, 'Who is this
that obscures my plans without knowledge?'
Surely I spoke of things I did not understand,
things too wonderful for me to know.
"You said, 'Listen now, and I will speak;
I will question you,
and you shall answer me.'
My ears had heard of you
but now my eyes have seen you.
Therefore I despise myself
and repent in dust and ashes."
Job 42.1-6

God is God and beyond that we need no answers or explanations. We may strive with our intellects to explore the nature of truth and there is nothing wrong with doing so; but God is beyond all this. He requires no justification, no explanation. Doctrine is a human endeavour. We spend a lot of time arguing about it; it divides Christians; it separates Christians from those of other faiths. God is to be worshipped not explained.

Can an experience that occurred when the brain was in a disordered state be real? I am not sure of the answer to that! The experience of the Divine has influenced my subsequent life and thought and for me it has been liberating and life enhancing. That must be important. As a neurologist I am reminded of the account of Prince Myshkin in Dostoyevsky's novel *The Idiot*. Like Dostoyevsky Myshkin had epilepsy; the type was temporal lobe epilepsy or what is now called complex partial seizures. These attacks may be associated with unusual experiences. Myshkin describes an ecstatic or mystical experience as a prelude to his seizure.

"He was thinking, incidentally, that there was a moment or two in his epileptic condition (if it occurred during the waking hours) almost before the fit itself when suddenly amid the sadness, spiritual darkness and depression, his brain seemed to catch fire at brief moments, and with an extraordinary momentum his vital forces were strained to the utmost all at once. His sensation of being alive and his awareness increased tenfold in these moments which flashed by like lightning. His mind and heart were flooded by a dazzling light. All his agitations, all his doubts and worries seemed composed in a twinkling, culminating in a great calm full of serene and harmonious joy and hope, full of understanding and the knowledge of the final cause. Reflecting about the moment afterwards, when he was well again, he often said to himself that all those gleams and flashes of the highest awareness and, hence, also of the 'highest mode of existence', were nothing but disease, a departure from the normal condition, and, if so, it was not at all the highest level of existence, but on the contrary, must be considered to be the lowest. And yet at last he arrived at the paradoxical conclusion. 'What if it is a disease?' he decided at last. 'What does it matter if it is an abnormal tension, if the result, if the moment of sensation, remembered and analysed in a state of health, turn out to be harmony and beauty brought to their highest state of perfection, and gives a feeling, undefined and undreamt-of till then, of completeness, proportion, reconciliation, and an ecstatic and prayerful fusion in the highest synthesis of life?"

We tend to be afraid of abnormality or extremes of human experience and behaviour. We are, in many respects, the victims of our brains. Although life experiences play an important part in what happens to us, some of us carry with us a constitution that makes us susceptible to clinical depression or epilepsy. The whole range of human experience must include these 'altered' states. We do not know enough to state with confidence that truth is only to be attained by those who comply with the prevailing concept of normality.

The greatest loss for the depressed person is hope and hope lies at the heart of Christianity. Hope is founded in a trust in the presence of a transcendent and mysterious God. The loss of hope is expressed in acts of attempted or successful self-destruction. Either life is meaningless and not worth living or it is so terrible that the agony of existence is far worse than the anonymity of death. This type of hopelessness is not the necessary accompaniment of extreme adversity. People at the edge of human existence, struggling for survival, may continue in that struggle despite everything, until the body becomes too weak to fight on. The disordered mind of the depressed person sees the world through 'a dark glass' and everything is centered on the self. The essential hope of Christianity is not self-centered. Hope is no hope at all if it depends on what happens to the individual.

Religion is frequently unfriendly towards those with abnormal states of mind. People who become depressed may be deemed to lack moral fibre, have weak faith, and be self-absorbed. Charitable and caring people may find it difficult to understand depression. Perhaps, this is because the mind is perceived as immune from disease. The separation of mind from brain also separates the mind from physical processes. The Bible has little to say about mental illness. It is possible that King Saul was rather more than jealous of David. His moods of 'jealous paranoia' could have been caused by mental illness. David played the harp for Saul and it seemed to relieve his mental anguish. The therapeutic value of music is now reasonably well established and this may well represent an early example of music therapy. Saul was harshly dealt with by God, and the Bible does not always make good reading for people in mental anguish.

Mathew 4.24 refers to Jesus healing people with diseases, including those who were possessed by devils and were lunatic. In Galatians 5.16–26 the writer describes and lists the fruit of the spirit. Peace and self-control indicate the possibility that such states are to be considered a feature of a life 'lived in the spirit' and that the opposite conditions are 'works of the flesh'. Those with mental illness may find it impossible to attain these levels of existence. Many Christians and adherents of other faiths are unable to control their minds when affected by serious mental illness.

The Bible refers to madness. Moses referred to it as arising from disobedience in Deuteronomy 38.34. Jesus appears to have been thought to be mad in Mark 3.21. Prophets were accused of madness in Hosea 9.7. But the Bible references are quite insufficient to come to any conclusions.

The lack of any worthwhile comments about depression or madness indicate that we cannot attempt to use scripture to guide us or advise us through the myriad of issues that exist in our world. Although a pre-modern culture may teach us some things, our current environment precludes using any biblical or sacred literature if it conflicts with the knowledge of a scientific and technological society.

Death

"Ay, but to die, and go we know not where;
To lie in cold abstraction, and to rot;"
Claudio in *Measure for Measure* by William Shakespeare

We do not experience our own deaths; our knowledge about death comes from observing the death of other humans and animals. Death is all around us. We become aware that we are part of all that is and not set over against it. Human awareness of death and thoughts about what may happen to us after death may be uniquely human, but they have evolved over aeons of time and it is not possible to pin point when this happened. We have extinct hominid cousins and perhaps they were developing a similar self-awareness of mortality to ourselves. Some animals may have levels of awareness that surprise us; the demarcation lines are not absolute. Although those with a religious disposition may link death with 'eternal life' this chapter deals with my experience of death through my work. This includes actively 'causing' death and letting people die. There is some reference to the concept of spirit and soul, as death exposes our difficulties in avoiding dualism.

The average life expectancy in Western Europe was 79 years for males and 84 years for females in 2017. The expectation is that these figures will increase. These are major changes to the situation prevailing one hundred and fifty years ago. Human life expectancy is not the longest in nature; other living organisms outlive us, but we are unique in having a conscious desire to live longer.

If we assume that life is good and worth living it is quite reasonable to be enthusiastic about longer life. Why should people die 'before their time' if it can be prevented? However, with our current state of medical knowledge greater age carries an increasing proneness to disease and difficulty with mobility and independent living. A major challenge in health care is to reduce disability and dependence in elderly people.

Most of us have a strong instinct to survive, and providing our balance of mind is intact, we prefer to be alive than dead. One only has to witness people on the edge of death through poverty and malnutrition to realise that life is not readily surrendered. Yet, there are situations when we may judge that the state of death is to be preferred to life regardless of beliefs about life after death. Examples that come to mind are people in a vegetative state, or situations where pain and suffering are so marked that it is felt inappropriate to strive officiously to keep alive.

The most obvious reaction to premature death by religious people in an era before modern medicine was:

"The Lord gave, and the Lord has taken away; may the name of the Lord be praised."

Job 1.21

This apparently passive response was a way of keeping oneself together and facing up to the reality of death. God was in control despite the random and meaningless loss of life. Meaninglessness was only at a human level because His ways were mysterious and beyond knowing. There seems to be nothing wrong with this approach, providing it does not feed passivity, and enforce a picture of God as a capricious figure who punishes people and their loved ones for obscure reasons.

Even today, we cannot blame people who take this approach when none of the advantages of modern life are available. Yet most of us are profoundly grateful to those who would not accept the inevitable and applied themselves to preventing premature death.

Human endeavour through medicine has achieved remarkable progress in 'conquering' death. The application of new knowledge has been irregular. Less affluent societies have not seen the same level of progress. Even in Western society there is a 'post code lottery'. Regulatory bodies may control access to new treatments because of cost criteria. We choose the paths of knowledge we wish to pursue, how we spend our lives and use our talents. Most of us would accept we have wasted much of our time and resources. How we direct our efforts in the creative process is a fundamental moral question. When God called humans to be stewards of creation, the implication was that we would use our abilities wisely, intuiting how we would spend our time and abilities. Despite achievements, we have failed much of the time.

We all have different experiences of death. It may not be that important to witness the moment of departure. Modern medicine has moved the definitions that we are familiar with. For the lay person death means the time when heart beat and respiration cease permanently. The overwhelming feature of death is that it represents the end of an individual organism. The body returns to dust. The individual we knew is no longer present in our world in a physical sense.

My first contact with human death was as a medical student beginning anatomy classes. We were divided into groups of six and allocated a body. These were the bodies of people, preserved in formalin, who had donated themselves after death to the medical school. Nowadays, anatomy is not taught in quite the same way. In those days each of us was to spend the best part of eighteen months dissecting the entire body. In the case of arms or legs there were three people to each limb. We shared the thorax and abdomen. We each spent one term on an individual brain.

Before the start of the anatomy course we were instructed that we should always treat the bodies with respect, being reminded of the great privilege we had been granted. Most of us were around eighteen years of age, very immature. Society had allowed us to do this on the understanding that we had been selected as 'Tomorrow's Doctors'. We did behave reasonably in the dissecting room. Our weekly ordeal in the viva voce on the particular work we were doing was the most demanding aspect of daily life. We stood or fell together. We could not pass on until we had satisfied our teachers that we had learned our anatomy. It was a very good introduction to teamwork!

There was no doubt that the bodies we were dissecting were dead. Although we did treat them with respect they were not people to us. We knew nothing of their past, their sorrows and joys. There was no narrative for us to connect with. Whatever animates and makes a human being live and seem a person was not present. Was this just because the heart was not beating, the chest moving, or something more? Was there some other presence, spirit, soul, that had departed and was elsewhere? One thing was certain; no 'conjuring tricks with bones' had taken place. Death was a real biological phenomenon, no different from any other animal death.

Another rather similar encounter with death was in the post mortem room. Each day in the medical school a list went up with details of the post mortem teaching sessions at lunchtime. We were meant to attend the room and one of the pathologists would carry out a teaching post mortem, seeking to discover the cause of death and giving us lessons in gross organ pathology. Some of the post mortems were on people dying in the adjacent hospital; others were involved in suicides or accidents in London. We were given a brief account of the medical history. Even this small detail provided a background or context for a life. The situation was different to the anatomy room. We were able to connect briefly with lives, although the reality of death was all around us.

After we moved to the hospitals as clinical students the experience of death broadened. The main hospital was near Trafalgar Square. People came there from a wide area, but there was a resident population nearby, many of whom were disadvantaged. We had many admissions from Bruce House, a local nightly lodging facility. People could have a bed there for a nominal amount. We soon got used to death from pneumonia. Was it a friend? Certainly, these were lives with apparently little to be happy about. We became aware of a sub-culture in the streets around us. This was a world that was remote from our own upbringings. Some of these deaths left one feeling guilty, uneasy and powerless. These were real people, but by the time we met them they were too sick to engage with.

We saw death in the operating theatre. These were the early days of cardiac surgery. As a student, there was no personal involvement, but later, working at a heart hospital as a house officer, I became very upset when people I had admitted died during or shortly after cardiac operations which now carry a very low mortality. These were people I had met and talked to. It was very different from the dissecting room. Working in a hospital gave death a sense of awfulness. It is hardly surprising that young doctors see death as a failure. It took a long time to understand that at times death is appropriate. It is sometimes better for someone to die than remain alive even when death is premature.

The death that distressed me most as a medical student was that of a young girl aged seven or eight years in East London. As part of our paediatric experience, we were attached to Shadwell Hospital in Stepney. The child was admitted in status epilepticus. This is continuous seizures without any recovery in between. Everyone fought to save her, but the seizures could not be controlled. I remember the feeling of devastation. There was a debate about what should have been done. Although I knew very little there was the feeling it should never have happened. The only life we know is this life. We should guard the lives of others as something precious. Saving life through better medicine was important. It was my first practical lesson in the need for medical specialisation, in this case neurology.

Many years later I was involved in deciding whether people in intensive care units (ITU) were brain dead or more specifically, brain stem dead. By this time, organ donation and transplant surgery had become part of medicine. A major source of organs was young people in Intensive Care Units with terminal brain damage from various causes. By then death was undergoing redefinition. Brain stem death was the recognised definition in the United Kingdom. This meant that if someone was in irreversible coma and the brain stem reflexes were absent on more than one occasion, over a specified period of time, they could be defined as being dead, providing the cause of this state was known and was not due to drugs. After discussion with the relatives, it was possible to turn off the respirator that was keeping them alive. If permission had been given, organs could be removed for transplantation. This would occur prior to withdrawing supportive treatment.

The difficulty about modern intensive care lies in the emergency treatment of people who are kept alive, but become profoundly impaired; some but not all will die at an early stage. We are unable to trust predictors of outcome sufficiently to allow them to die in peace. The need for transplants has created a situation that requires harvesting of organs before the respirator is turned off. From one perspective, this reduces death to a biological debate. However, providing the individual is treated with respect as an end in his or her self and not a means, there is no moral harm to that person. Whatever the soul or spirit is, one is not killing it by such actions. If the soul dies with the mind it is already absent. If the soul is an immaterial immortal part of us it cannot be killed.

The difficulty that some may have with the act of turning off a respirator is that it appears to be an act of killing someone rather than letting die. However, if it is accepted that the person is already dead it cannot be active euthanasia. Further, the patient would not be breathing without technology. There is a huge difference between actively trying to kill a person and letting them die.

Although I deal with suffering elsewhere, it is relevant in discussing whether severe suffering ever allows the possibility of promoting actions hastening death. Allowing human suffering to continue is very difficult. Suffering is commonly linked with pain and a familiar model is the person with terminal cancer. Pain is an important physical aspect of human suffering, but there are other aspects often given less prominence. Mental deterioration and severe muscle weakness are not accompanied inevitably by pain. Breathlessness at rest is very unpleasant, but it would not usually be associated with the word pain. In one sense, all suffering is mental because it is the reaction of a mind to a particular circumstance. If we did not have brains, we could not suffer. It is mental awareness that is the key factor.

I became aware of issues surrounding euthanasia when involved in the care of someone with Huntington's chorea, an inherited brain disease that causes unpleasant involuntary movements and progressive dementia. I knew the person, Ralph, well. He had been an executive in a flourishing company and had travelled extensively. At the time in question he was in a tragic state, demented but not without some periods of insight. He was in hospital with a chest infection. He was given antibiotics. His wife came to see me and it was quite clear that she would much prefer that her husband died. The whole situation was intolerable. Because of behavioural difficulties Ralph was already on sedative drugs. I was asked to increase them with a view to hastening death. Initially I did so, thinking that increasing the dose was justified to relieve mental anguish, even if death ensued. However, there was no physical deterioration and it became clear that only a definite lethal dose of some agent would cause death at this point. I knew I could not do that and reduced the medication, after which Ralph lived for a good number of years in a pathetic state.

It is naïve to consider that human suffering can be relieved in all circumstances. This is at the core of the argument in favour of euthanasia. If your much-loved dog is in a terminal distressed state, you put her out of her misery. Why not humans, particularly if they ask us to do so?

There are no easy answers to this question unless we use the Ten Commandments. 'Thou shall not kill' is clear enough. But there is a difference between killing and letting die. In contrast to the situation with Ralph it is important not to strive officiously to keep alive in every circumstance. These decisions are never easy and are not the exclusive domain of doctors, nurses or relatives. The subject of the decision may be in a position to give a clear opinion or have provided a 'Living Will' prior to the illness.

Bill had had a very severe head injury. He had minimal or no awareness; he had severe paralysis and could do nothing for himself. He came from the centre of a northern town and belonged to a close-knit community. His brother and sister-in-law were determined to care for him after he was discharged from the rehabilitation unit. He was fed by gastrostomy tube and was subject to recurrent chest infections that required hospital admission on a regular basis.

His relatives used to sit him outside the front door in the street of terraced houses in a wheelchair. There was no evidence that he was aware of his surroundings, but he was well known and people would greet him as they passed. During one admission with pneumonia I sat down with the relatives to discuss whether it was appropriate to give Bill repeated courses of antibiotics. I was hoping that they would indicate that Bill's quality of life was so poor that it was wrong to keep him alive. Their response was different. They told me that they wanted him to have the best possible life and that they were committed to this. This meant for them that he should get the best possible treatment and this included treating every infection.

Although I had severe reservations about their viewpoint I did not feel that it was right to make it an issue. I could have argued that acting on behalf of Bill's interests a neutral person might have considered that the state of death was to be preferred to life. It cannot be assumed that relatives always act in the best interests of a loved one.

I use this example to stress that even allowing people to die can be a contentious subject. Examples that have come to the courts in recent years have involved decisions about whether it is permissible to withdraw supportive treatment from people in catastrophically impaired states, often on respirators. In individual cases, it has been ruled permissible to turn off the respirator, cease tube feeding and basic nutrition, allowing death to occur. As has been mentioned, the existence of this situation usually stems from initial high technology intervention. Although common sense might suggest that decisions about letting people die need to be taken, the acceptance of death remains a major problem.

At the core of much traditional Christian thinking is the idea that death is something that requires 'conquering'. Jesus 'conquered' death and rose to new life. Death therefore is not to be feared because of the possibility of eternal life. I do not want to dwell on eternal life at this stage, but raise the question whether it is appropriate to see death as an enemy regardless of beliefs. It is legitimate to 'conquer' or prevent premature death by medical advance, but this must have limitations. The idea that death is an enemy unless there is 'eternal life' is understandable in the presence of unmerited suffering, and also as a way of being united with loved ones, but that does not justify the word 'conquer'.

Many would argue that death is a necessity to allow creation to unfold. If the world were full of very old people and animals, there would be a reduced opportunity to explore creative possibilities, present in each succeeding generation. Our complex ecological systems are distorted by excessive meddling with the natural environment. Longevity is likely to increase further in many countries, but life will remain finite. Even modest increases in longevity will place a huge strain on resources.

Death is part of life. It may be premature and due to disaster or disease, but in ideal circumstances it gives life shape. It is something to accept and be grateful for.

Recently I heard a brief discussion between an academic scientist and an Anglican curate. Much of the debate centered on creationism versus evolution. But at one point the curate pointed out that for him, as a Christian, death is a problem that requires 'conquering'. In what sense did Jesus conquer death? He faced up to death, premature death. Although he was subject to the normal human reluctance to die an unnecessary death, it happened because he was determined to maintain integrity. He did not place the saving of his life above the message he had come to preach. One can argue that this is a central feature of his victory over death. Eternal life is another issue.

Postponing the moment of death, regardless of the quality of life, can be a distortion of life itself. Death is treated as an end to be avoided at all costs.

I recall the distressing example of a lady with Creutzfeldt-Jakob disease, a rapid form of progressive dementia and severe physical disability caused by a prion infection. Her condition deteriorated rapidly and she passed in to an unresponsive vegetative state. She was artificially fed and kept alive at all costs for over a year. The nursing staff found this very distressing. Her husband was adamant that his wife should not be allowed to die.

Any sign of infection resulted in an insistence that maximum medication was given. He was suspicious and even paranoid about staff attitudes. He was completely unwilling to entertain the possibility that death for his wife was a release. Fortunately, before the inevitable legal conflict developed his wife did die of an uncontrolled pneumonia.

Accepting the inevitability of death, and the appropriateness of allowing some to die, does not necessarily justify killing people who 'suffer', even if someone makes the request. Attitudes to life may determine our attitudes to death. If life is a gift, not a right or commodity, it is reasonable to ponder whether it is justified to terminate life by a deliberate act. The 'slippery slope' argument is based on the fear that acts of killing will not be restricted to people suffering in terminal states. The community might lose with the introduction of widespread active euthanasia. It is certainly vital that health care workers are trusted and seen as agents who always place the wellbeing of their patient first. Multiple murders by a medical practitioner in the United Kingdom drew attention to the complexity of giving any role in relation to killing to doctors. It would be very easy to confuse murder and euthanasia. The general public should be justifiably concerned about the boundaries of legitimate activity involving doctors and nurses. Common sense is a sound theological position, and that suggests that we should never give the health care professions a formal role in terminating life.

Although we may expect life expectancy to increase, particularly in areas where it is currently well below levels in developed countries, there is no evidence that the human species could live forever. Our planet has finite resources and there is no reason to believe that extreme longevity is desirable. Novels such as *After Many a Long Summer* by Aldous Huxley have explored the quest for the elixir for 'living for ever'. Whether it is essence of carp or any other substance it is not a necessary route to happiness. It is better to accept death, not as an enemy but a part of our finite existence; as part of creation.

Resurrection

"He who binds to himself a joy does the winged life destroy;
but he who kisses the joy as it flies lives in eternity's sunrise."
William Blake

*He had experienced several occasions when he was aware for a
short while of feelings that were not temporal. Certainly, they
were linked with temporal circumstance, but somehow, they
transcended these and hinted of a quality of life beyond the
ordinary.*

*One such experience went back to childhood – the occasion
when his mother drove him in the English countryside after an
eye operation and he was acutely aware of the light filtering
through beech and oak along Sussex lanes. The physical
experience evoked something beyond it, intimations of joy and
beauty that were timeless and deeply reassuring.*

*There were similar experiences evoked by different events,
but having a common quality. He could recall the remarkable
sense of release and new life walking along the Sussex beach
promenade after his illness in India.*

*An experience coincided with Easter one year. Ten days
before this he had been on a philosophy weekend in Wales with
a medical colleague. The first night away he was awakened by a
rigor. His body was shaking and he felt very unwell. He was
aware of perineal pain. It did not take long to realise he had some*

form of acute infection involving the prostate. He managed to get to the night porter who contacted his friend. It was decided to make for home. The friend, mistakenly filling his car with diesel fuel stalled the journey and it was necessary to wait shivering under a blanket while the friend's mother, who lived in Wales, came to the rescue! Eventually they returned to the North of England. He took antibiotics, but there was no improvement and his muscles became weaker.

On Maundy Thursday, he was admitted to the neurological ward and investigation revealed a prostate abscess. He was transferred to the adjacent hospital for surgery. He asked the surgeon if the operation could be avoided. He was given a firm answer in the negative. He waited on the Good Friday to go to the operating theatre. The anaesthetist declined to give him a general anaesthetic and the procedure was done under spinal anaesthesia. When the pus was released into the circulation from the abscess the upper non-paralysed part of his body began to shake.

On return to the ward he remained in a paralysed state waiting for the next day, return of movement and an improved sense of wellbeing. By Saturday he had entered into a state of calm. He was acutely aware of the care of the nurses, their good humour and skill. He became aware of an inexpressible sensation of release. Everything seemed very good. Being aware had an exquisite tinge to it. On Sunday, young people came from a nearby church and wheeled him in a chair to the hospital chapel for the Easter Day service. There was another beginning. Life was a treasure. There was the possibility of a new start. Subsequently, he changed his job and life orientation. Although it was painful, he turned away from the situation that was stifling him and experienced huge relief.

People experience many kinds of special moments that evoke extra-temporal glimpses of reassurance and joy. Marcel Proust describes his own in the last novel of *A La Researche du Temps Perdu:*

"Why had the images of Combray, at these two different moments, given me a joy which was like a certainty and which I understood clearly that what the sensation of the uneven paving stones, the stillness of the napkin, the taste of the Madeleine had awakened in me had no connection with what I frequently tried to recall to myself of Venice, Balbec, Combray, with the help of an undifferentiated memory; and I understood that the reason why life may be judged to be trivial although at certain moments it appears to be so beautiful is that we form our judgement, ordinarily, on the evidence not of life itself but of those quite different images which preserve nothing of life…"

For Proust, these special moments were resurrections. He uses this word. For him beyond the ordinary, the descriptions of life, lay an extra-temporal reality. It was the work of all art and music to go beyond the surface and uncover the eternal.

It is difficult to speak of moral quality in such experiences; they appear to transcend morality. The quality of such realisations is what might be described as new life or true life. It is what most of us just glimpse. It is different to the understanding of eternal life that is one of the pre-occupations of Christianity. We need to balance our thoughts about 'resurrections' in this life and the possibility of some form of life after death. The difficulty with the latter is that lies beyond rationality and conceptual thinking. The word 'eternal' has no meaning beyond 'space-time'.

One cannot ignore the preoccupation with life after death that has occurred across many cultures over vast tracts of time. Egyptian funereal custom certainly assumed some kind of material life after death. The traditional Jewish view, prior to the Maccabees, was that resurrection did not happen; the dead went to a shadowy Sheol. The understanding of this word is difficult. Initially, it appeared to be a place where all went regardless of righteousness. It was a place where nothing happened. Later the word Hades was borrowed from Greek tradition and the concept developed as a place of waiting for all, prior to judgment. Those deemed righteous would be restored with a heavenly body. The damned would be tortured by their own sins. The word Hell became linked with the abode of the damned.

Although souls, spirit and people are mentioned elsewhere, their presence in Christian tradition influences our understanding of resurrection profoundly. We cling to these words amidst biological decay. It is a matter of observation that physical disintegration of the brain is related to impaired mental function. Mind and brain are intimately connected. The nature of the connection is a matter for philosophical debate. At one extreme is the materialist view that brain equals mind. All mental attributes are neurochemical and neurophysiological phenomena. There is no separate immaterial entity of mind. The possibility of some form of eternal life has been explored by two philosopher/theologians, John Hick and Hans Kung. Hick in his book *Death and Eternal life* explores the subject in Western and Eastern traditions. He comes to tentative positive conclusions about the possibility of eternal life. The difficulty with his approach is that he appears to separate mind from brain. Although this is a legitimate viewpoint I do not think it supported by neuroscience. Kung's conclusions in *Eternal life?* are vague. One thing he dismisses is the value of near death experiences.

A different way of expressing the brain-mind problem is to regard mind as an emergent level of existence, dependant on brain, but not reducible to neurochemistry. A different language is required to express mind. But it is another matter altogether to claim that mind is something non-material that can exist without the brain substance.

A good deal of Christian thinking about the concepts of soul and spirit assumes that these are immaterial entities that exist independently of the body. This dualist philosophy implies that there is a 'ghost in the machine', quite separate from our material selves. The idea that the soul enters the body at a particular point, for example at fertilisation, implantation or 'quickening' is impossible to refute. But it is very difficult for someone exposed to the harsh reality of human brain pathology to accept dualism.

Lady Helen Oppenheimer in her book *Looking Before and After* suggests that the term soul may be used to describe the potential for an emergent identity that is spiritual in the sense that the soul is the focus of what is best in humanity. Therefore, we could be relatively soulless because the shape and nature of our lives will determine the development of our soul. This does not imply that soul is a separate element in our make-up, but an integral part of our being.

Belief in an immaterial soul makes it easier for people to come to terms with eternal life. If the soul departs the body at death one can imagine a future existence either disembodied or clothed in an immortal body.

Plato certainly seems to have placed very little emphasis on the body and his devaluing of the non-mental has had a deleterious effect on Christian thinking. The body is seen by some as a threat to the spiritual, something that has to be subjugated and controlled so that the mind is freed for higher pursuits. Some of Pauline theology may be understood as denigrating the physical.

Helen Oppenheimer summarises the problems many Christians have with the soul by pointing out that Christians have always found it difficult to extricate themselves from dualism. They feel readily threatened by the concept of basic wholeness and integrity of the human person. The idea of the soul as a separate entity is deeply reassuring. Without it there is a risk that we are material beings without spiritual natures. Yet, without the recognition of our wholeness of being we are avoiding facing reality. We are reluctant to acknowledge souls in animals explicitly because we consider ourselves special. Separating ourselves from other organisms is misguided. We are as much part of evolutionary nature as any other living entity.

Some of this will be referred to in the chapter on persons. The point here is that this concept does not accord with the traditional Jewish view of humans as psychosomatic entities. Pauline theology suggests also that resurrection includes the whole being, not a disembodied mind.

Limitations in human language have led to difficulty and much confusion in describing the resurrection experience, but there is no denying that life after death is a core part of traditional Christianity. Arguments either way on the subject have been a 'stumbling block' for many people·

The famous assertion by Bishop Jenkins that the Resurrection is not a 'conjuring trick with bones' may seem to be stating the obvious, but it caused an uproar. One supposes that it really upset some people to have the suggestion that the 'empty tomb', at best, did not matter, and at worst was a serious impediment to the proper understanding of resurrection. An empty tomb implies that Jesus got up and walked away. The time frame was too short to allow total decay. But that implies resuscitation not resurrection.

We are part of material creation and at death return to become part of the total mystery of the universe. We are just like any other animal in that respect. The resuscitation of a dead body is not consistent with being part of material creation, and in the case of Jesus, being a human. Therefore, there appears to be confusion in describing an empty tomb. The appearance of a resurrected Jesus to Mary Magdalene describes a totally different experience, not dependent on an empty tomb. The body was not material in the ordinary sense of that word and could not be touched. The experience is beyond the normal range of human language. The language used is poetic and metaphorical. There is a marked divergence of opinion within Christianity about resurrection. This is exemplified in the debate between the theologians Marcus Borg and Tom Wright. Borg understands resurrection as a metaphor; he sees the truth of Easter as grounded in the Christian experience of Jesus as a living spiritual reality in the present. Wright explores it from an historical literal perspective and insists that what happened to bring Christianity into being was more concrete than that. My own personal view is that Wright does not take account of the cultural setting of the time, and his view depends on an interventionist model of God that I have rejected elsewhere.

If we reduce resurrection to something historical that can be 'handled', we impair the essential mystery of life; we ignore the limitations of our brains that are locked into a restricted view of ultimate reality. We do not know what relationship our 'reality' has to ultimate truth. Science provides explanatory models that assist us in functioning in the world but, we do not know the status of our science. The same applies to theology. We have to allow the rich variety of understandings of God and the world to stand together while espousing our own preferences.

Why does one want to believe in life after death? Loss is a pervasive feature of human existence. We find loss very difficult to come to terms with. Loss of loved ones, loss of health and strength, our own extinction, are human features. On our riverbank at home we had eight geese. Most years they bred unsuccessfully. The eggs were washed away in the floodwater as the river rose and fell. Even if goslings were hatched the death rate was very high. Stoats, the local pike, foxes, accounted for most of them. The geese just carried on; they seemed unperturbed by these awful setbacks. They did not appear to respond to loss; yet we are aware that dogs and whales grieve. There is evidence that a sense of loss is not restricted to Homo sapiens.

As I have mentioned elsewhere the premature loss of loved ones was commonplace before modern medicine. The belief that there was another existence that made up for a short and brutal life allowed some level of future hope. Mothers died in childbirth. Infant mortality and child death were an everyday reality. There was little expectation that the ravages of disease would be conquered. The world was a savage place. Heaven was a place where earth's sorrows were washed away. There would be no more crying. life on earth was seen as a temporary sojourn on the way to something better.

The argument was that all injustice and unmerited suffering would be transformed. The debate for and against this model were rehearsed famously in Dostoyevsky's great novel *The Brothers Karamazov*. Ivan is quite unable to accept that unmerited injustice and suffering can be made up for by eternal bliss. Aloyisha takes the opposite view. Ivan's basic argument is that the world requires changing if one can ever accept the idea of a loving God who cares for individuals.

He uses the example of a retired general who had extensive lands and two thousand serfs. He had hundreds of hounds and a hundred mounted whips. A serf boy threw a stone that accidentally struck the paw of the general's favourite hound. The general took the boy and locked him up. The following morning, he released him and made him run, setting the hounds and whips on him in front of his mother. The hounds tore him to pieces.

Ivan uses children to focus his argument:

"Listen: if all have to suffer so as to buy eternal harmony by their suffering what have children to do with it – tell me please…

For you see, Aloyisha, it may really happen that if I live to that moment, or rise again to see it, I shall perhaps cry aloud with the rest, as I look at the mother embracing the child's torturer: 'Thou art just O lord!' But I do not want to cry aloud then…

And if the sufferings of children go to make up the sum of sufferings which is necessary for the purchase of truth, then I say beforehand that the entire truth is not worth such a price."

This problem of evil has no answers. Rewards and compensation in heaven may reassure if we have the faith to believe this. If God does not exist there is no problem. Everything can be put down to the lottery of existence. Matters can only improve through human endeavour and morality. On the other hand, if God does exist, He is either deeply mysterious in his purposes which will be revealed in the fullness of time, or there is an evil force in the world that battles God; Satan, the Devil. Many religions have struggled to explain evil in the world and the simplest solution is to posit an opposite pole to a loving God. The Bible certainly refers to evil on this basis, including demon or satanic possession; but combines this with the possibility of human choice. Zoroastrianism and Manichaeism use the dualism of good and evil to explain our world. Nowadays there has been a decline in the belief in a personal devil. An understanding of evil is made easier if Satan exists.

Dostoyevsky was specifically debating aspects of suffering using the example of gross human evil. The great importance of his exploration is that neither knowledge nor scientific progress reduces suffering in the end, only love properly applied. No amount of heavenly bliss makes up for a lifetime of suffering if one agrees with Ivan.

Another reason for wanting to believe in eternal life is to know God more fully, to see God 'face to face'. There is an element in most of us that longs for contact with the ultimate source of our being. We recognise ourselves as creatures, but we desire to transcend our human limitation and know God. If I understand the book of Job that does not imply that we have explanations. That is a very human failing. Job saw God and that was all he needed.

Knowing God is about quality of existence. It has absolutely nothing to do with living forever. It is not something to be defined in space and time or any conceivable mode of existence.

We must even ask ourselves whether such an experience has anything to do with the ego we link with ourselves. The abolition of desire is at the core of Eastern spirituality and is present in Christian tradition. How realistic this is, in the face of human biology, may be debatable, but it is impossible to deny the importance of the tradition. The Buddha story describes a man that was able to overcome desire and find enlightenment. Jesus similarly did not seek to save his life but found it in giving it up for the cause he served.

The implication of this is that true life, eternal life, is not measured in time or continued existence, it is pure essence, and one cannot locate it. Resurrection, as Harry Williams suggested in his book *True Resurrection,* is not something reserved for death of the body. We do not need to worry about what happens to us when we die. Far too much of our thinking about eternal life is negative.

It is quite impossible for the human brain to live in an extra-temporal world continuously. We may have glimpses of quality that have been described. We cannot know what will happen to us. Crude pictures of what it is like may comfort us, but it is important that we do not impose this on others who think and feel differently. Human life is many faceted and lived at different levels. It is unwise to expect everyone to live with the same images. It can be argued that the test of any great religion is a capacity to engage people at many levels of understanding. A religion such as Hinduism may appear to vary from a sophisticated philosophical structure to crude village polytheism, but it embraces all types of people at their differing levels of knowledge and temperament. Christianity has the capacity to do the same but is severely hampered by the cult of 'orthodoxy'.

Mother Julian summarised how we should look at our future: "All will be well and all manner of things shall be well." That is all we need. But that is not a saying that can be spoken of tritely. It is the kind of truth won after a lifetime of exploration.

Suffering

"He sat in a wheeled chair, waiting for dark,
And shivered in his ghastly suit of grey,
Legless, sewn short at elbow. Through the park
Voices of boys rang saddening like a hymn,
Voices of play and pleasure after day,
Till gathering sleep had mothered them from him."
Wilfred Owen from *Disability*

We use the word suffering a great deal, perhaps far too much. We say someone suffers from migraine, indigestion, multiple sclerosis. We could just state that they have these conditions. Perhaps we want to express in a clumsy way that we realise their lot is far worse than ours. We could be stating we are aware that they are going through mental anguish because that is the essential nature of human suffering.

Pain is a sensation originating in peripheral receptors in our body and entering consciousness as pain at the level of the thalamic nuclei of the brain and the cerebral cortex. Pain warns us of danger although the cause may be trivial. However, pain does not equal suffering. We suffer when awareness of pain is linked with other parts of the brain, particularly the limbic system that has an important role in our emotional reactions. Suffering is a mental, emotional response to a whole range of circumstances, not necessarily physically painful. The essential response of the sufferer is that he/she is distressed by what is happening. There is a strong desire for the cause of the suffering to be removed, but a powerlessness to alter the situation alone.

The capacity for suffering varies enormously. Apart from our own genetic makeup that governs our personalities, expectations and cultural environment have a major impact. In a situation where people have very high expectations about health and quality of life even minor adversity may cause mental anguish.

Suffering is not necessarily concerned with our own predicaments. We suffer when those whom we care for are ill or distressed in any way. We suffer when our pet animals die. We are capable of suffering when we witness directly or even indirectly, through the media, the plight of others far removed from our world. This may drive us to action aimed at helping relieve this suffering.

The suffering that concerns us most is that which is unmerited. It is obvious that a great deal of human suffering is brought about by human behaviour. The picture drawn by Wilfred Owen at the head of this chapter is a stark reminder of the terrors of war. We have a great propensity to harm each other and ourselves. It is quite possible to make the resources of the world available on a more equitable basis and reduce the burden of starvation and disease in developing countries. We do not need to damage our bodies with substances we know to be harmful.

However, at the end of all this human-initiated suffering there is a hard core of suffering due to disease and natural disaster that seems difficult to prevent. It seems impossible to avoid the natural response of emotional distress at the death of loved ones.

One concludes that humans are born to suffer although the level of suffering is not evenly distributed.

I recall meeting a lady whose husband had been lost at sea; not long after her son developed a malignant brain tumour and she came to see me with symptoms that were diagnosed as multiple sclerosis. Most of us can recall similar examples of the uneven distribution of suffering.

Why should this happen? That is the straightforward question to which there is no answer that fully satisfies. As far as we know these things are built in to the fabric of our universe and human endeavour does not have the means to prevent them or put them right. Human progress has certainly made a difference to the burden of disease, but it continues; previous generations have known appalling suffering.

Patterns of disease have changed in many parts of the world. But it is incorrect to state that the great infections have been eliminated. We place great emphasis on genetic disease. This is partly because there is hope that the greater understanding of genetics will result in the successful treatment of many diseases, including cancer and infections. However, it would be naïve to conclude that the cure of all human diseases lies around the corner.

There is a tendency to link suffering with illness and disease in the context of a medical model. Even the Church's healing ministry over-emphasises medical illness. From a theological perspective, it seems that suffering in the world is fundamentally about alienation, from God and each other. Any worthwhile concept of healing is certainly concerned with reducing suffering, but this is achieved through integration. This involves accepting, in a constructive way, situations that exist, that cannot be removed. Medicine does have a role in reducing human suffering, but the mere treatment of disease or providing supportive therapy and services for those with incurable and progressive disorders is only a partial solution.

The Bible provides accounts of people having their suffering relieved through the action of Jesus. Jesus, for Christians, provides an example of engagement in the world for the benefit of others, but to take his 'healing' miracles as examples of divine intervention is mistaken. To regard Jesus as a 'miracle worker', authenticating his divine status is a theological error. A careful reading of the Bible will reveal that Jesus did not wish to emphasise the miraculous. As I have indicated elsewhere, a pre-modern culture interpreted events differently. There were many miraculous healers at that time. In Mark's Gospel Peter proclaims Jesus as Messiah. He is told to avoid proclaiming it. This is sometimes referred to as the Messianic secret. Some commentators do not consider that this had anything to do with secrecy, but that Peter had proclaimed Jesus for the wrong reasons. His acclamation was based on miracle working and the picture of Jesus as a triumphant Messiah in the Davidic tradition. That ignored that the path Jesus was to take was *The Way of the Cross.* This was the antithesis of miracle working. Jesus may have had a sense of what might occur as a result of his ministry; but regardless of this, Peter had distorted the nature of what Jesus was about. Each Gospel writer had a purpose. Mark wrote from the perspective of someone who knew that Jesus had suffered. Peter had yet to understand this. It should be noted that Peter used the word Messiah in Mark. The words 'Son of God' are not used.

Much pious literature has been written on the subject of Jesus' suffering. We are called to meditate on his suffering and journey with him through *Holy Week*. But what do we mean by it? If we look at the physical suffering of Jesus we may well be prompted to ask in what way was it worse than the experiences of many others exposed to disease, torture and execution? This cannot be measured; but it is clear that many people have suffered appallingly. It is not enough to state that the uniqueness of Jesus' suffering was because it was unmerited. Other good people have suffered in this way.

Surely someone will say, if Jesus was the Son of God he would have suffered less than most because of whom he was. One feature of Gnosticism was a claim that as Jesus was not really human, he never suffered as the Son of God. One of the great debates in early Christianity was the nature of Jesus. There were attempts to explain how he could be both divine and human. Monophysitism is the view or teaching that Christ had only one nature, either entirely divine, or, in some versions, a seamless blend of human and divine such that the two were inseparable. This presents a problem, because if Jesus had one nature his suffering is meaningless and the doctrine of the atonement fails. The atonement is rescued by dyophysitism. Dyophysitism is the doctrine that Christ had two distinct natures in one person, united and in perfect harmony, but nevertheless separate and distinct. This allowed Jesus to suffer. Monophysitism was rejected at the council of Chalcedon. However, Eastern Oriental Orthodox Churches retained it, while Western and mainstream Orthodox Churches refuted it. These doctrines are unhelpful, tortuous, and disconnected from modern thought. It is best to regard Jesus as a man who suffered. If we wish to promote his divine status we can regard him as being full of the spirit of God. One of the problems of Christology is being consistent about Jesus' humanity and deciding whether it is in any way possible to hold to his divinity at the same time.

It is certainly important to emphasise that in working out any point of contact between the suffering of Jesus and the rest of us we need to believe that he was a human being, a man. He therefore had a human brain, human thoughts and human emotions. His body worked in the same way as anyone else. Because we know very little about Jesus there is a great temptation to evade his humanity. It is easier not to think about mundane human things when worshipping someone as a god. There is considerable difficulty in steering the right course between Jesus the man and one who is worshipped as Lord. Many people seem unwilling to face up to the consequences of Jesus' humanity. Unwittingly he is seen as a god dressed up in human clothing, someone who knows everything. The idea of Jesus' sinless nature is confusing unless we can understand this as a symbol of his relationship to God. In a similar way that the Buddha was able to overcome desire and achieve Nibbana, Jesus overcame love of his own life for its own sake and found union with God.

Jesus probably suffered great mental anguish when he realised that the message he preached was not widely welcomed or understood. He was, we are told, betrayed by a friend and put to death. He remained true to his message. He overcame the temptation to opt out. He suffered, possibly because he saw his mission falling apart, his vision unfulfilled. He was abandoned.

Suffering is closely linked with abandonment. We are sustained in our personal ordeals by the love of others. Jesus was sustained and achieved integration through his relationship to

God, but he is recorded as saying, "My God, My God, why have you forsaken me?"

We think of Jesus as a person who cared and loved others regardless of status and position. He gave himself for the cause of the Kingdom. The importance of his suffering lies in his rejection and abandonment, the rejection of good in favour of evil.

Jesus makes us aware of the awfulness of attempting to destroy good. We are reminded that whatever the appearances, good cannot be destroyed; evil will not triumph ultimately. But we do have to live with our diseases, our wounds. Those who forget this seriously distort the whole picture of suffering. The practical importance of this for the world of human disease is the importance of accepting the situation; paradoxically we reduce our suffering by making it part of who we are, and by doing so, reduce it. We learn to cope better.

We recognise that abandonment of others is something that intensifies suffering. This does not mean that we talk incessantly to our friends who suffer, swamping them with platitudes and kindness. We can show solidarity by learning how to be there, to be still with them, and stand with them. It makes an enormous difference.

It is important for us to avoid self-absorption. When something bad happens to us it is commonplace to become inward looking and cease to look outwards at all. The hallmark of Jesus' life was concern for others, particularly those in need. We are greatly helped if we can maintain interest in the lives of others. Integration is not about prolonged 'umbilical' gazing! We need to make a journey inward to keep in touch with our feelings and our thoughts but we reduce our suffering and aid our healing by looking outwards. Our suffering is helped if we can remain engaged with the world.

Can others adsorb or absorb the distress of the sufferer? It is possible. The image of the *'wounded healer'* may apply to Jesus or us. Liberation theology includes the identification of Jesus with the dispossessed, the one who identifies and absorbs some of the suffering of those without an advocate. In a similar manner, if one is able to stand close to someone who suffers, some of that distress may be adsorbed on to the surface of oneself or absorbed into one's being.

I saw a young man in an outpatient clinic. I had seen him on several previous occasions, but he had frequently failed to attend. He had the progressive neurological disorder known as Huntington's chorea. This disease produces unpleasant and disabling involuntary movements which interrupt purposeful activity and interfere with basic functions such as walking, manual dexterity, feeding, swallowing and speech. Alongside this, most people with Huntington's chorea undergo a progressive intellectual deterioration, and there is often associated behavioural disorder, including increased aggression. People with the disease have an increased risk of suicide. The young man had a relationship with a young woman and there were two children in the family. Although he had an emotional attachment to his girlfriend, he was unable to live with her because he could no longer control his behaviour. This distressed him.. He had been under the care of a psychiatrist and there was social worker involvement. He was already on medication for his involuntary movements, but it was making little difference. Several days after seeing me he committed suicide by hanging himself.

I think that example demonstrates the powerlessness, loss of control and destruction of identity that are important features of a progressive disorder. It is a good example of unmerited suffering. It raises the issue that although this young man's brain was severely damaged he had the insight to suffer and was aware of his awful predicament. The powerlessness extended to those who were onlookers; this can lead to an avoidance of contact because we are unsure how we can help.

The subsequent isolation is an important aspect of suffering. Some people have such an overwhelming feeling of isolation, even when surrounded by others. They want to be on their own, away from people they know, as they think it will cause less pain and embarrassment to all concerned. It is extremely difficult to absorb this kind of suffering but not impossible.

A lady with multiple sclerosis told me of such feelings. She found it increasingly difficult to feel part of her home and church community. Everyone was very well meaning but she felt she was losing her own identity and that it was time to give up and live in an anonymous environment.

Progressive disabling conditions are very distressing to those observing the deterioration in bodily and mental function. When the setting is a supportive family there is a familiar framework for the local community to link up with, but this is not always the case. We need to face up to the destructive nature of progressive disability on family life. Families do disintegrate and the serious stresses that are placed on the family are a challenge to our communities.

The example of the young man with Huntington's chorea was a difficult one. Unless we surround ourselves with 'walls of concrete' we are bound to be troubled about issues such as the nature of personhood. We may be strongly attracted to the idea of putting people beyond their suffering. I remember the reaction of an ordinand on one of our summer schools after a visit to a psycho-geriatric unit. He was quite honest. He did not see those there as people and thought euthanasia an entirely appropriate option. It was difficult to know whether his reaction was largely related to his own inability to cope with reality or a genuine concern for the people in the unit.

In the Christian tradition, as in others, human beings are thought to be created in the image of God, and however dire the situation, many uphold this belief. We may worry about the silence of God in these situations, but that is usually a reflection of our own silence and lack of involvement. We may ask the question why we place people with the same kind of condition in special units. Our tendency to distance and institutionalise some people is a challenge to our social structures. We place the suffering of the world at a safe distance and hope others will deal with it.

It is a reasonable principle to look at some of the worst-case scenarios before we get too complacent about some of the solutions we offer. How do we incorporate someone like the young man into our religious and local communities? How do we absorb and share his suffering? There are no easy solutions but faced with the marred image of God we are challenged to come alongside such people and discover what ministry they have for us. If we believe that all God's creation ministers to us than there can be no exceptions. How do we avoid regarding people with severe and progressive disabilities as people to be cared for and looked after, but without any distinctive and worthwhile ministry of their own? People with minimal potential, passive sufferers. It is very easy to avoid the effort involved in discovering new roles for people in this situation. It is easier to 'retire' them and look after them. Whether we are referring to the clergy or the lay person we often find it difficult to monitor change, remaining unaware of the grief and anguish that result from a loss of role and purpose.

The hope is that our communities allow those with progressive and often severe disabilities to be part of us; allowed to witness with us and to us. Even when we can see little that they can accomplish we must acknowledge and accept them as they are, for they mirror what we might have been or may become. We reduce suffering through true community.

I have described elsewhere this sense of community described movingly in Vincent Donovan's book *The Rediscovery of Christianity*. He discovers among the Masai of East Africa communal living and believing unfamiliar to Western Christianity. In this community as the Headman Ndangoya pointed out everyone is part of the whole, whoever they are.

Souls and People

"No civilized society can thrive upon victims, whose humanity has been permanently mutilated."
Rabindranath Tagore

At the core of this discussion is the issue of how we treat each other. Whether we talk about persons or souls we enter difficult territory. It is much easier to use these words than come to an agreement about what they mean. It is the case that the use of the word person avoids the religious disagreements about the meaning of soul. As discussed earlier I am not aware of any coherent definition of a separate soul that stands up to critical scrutiny, but one cannot avoid some consideration of the word as it has been used to bolster arguments as to when something becomes a person, and this is relevant in a discussion of how we treat members of our species at the various stages of life. The idea of the soul as an immaterial entity has bedevilled theological discourse.

The Bible does not engage in major philosophical debates. There is some evidence of the influence of Greek philosophical ideas in parts of the New Testament such as John's Gospel. Greek philosophy was brought to bear on the nature of Jesus in this book, but there is no comprehensive investigation of the meaning of the words soul and spirit or the word person.

Judaism regards the human being as a psychosomatic entity in the image of God and traditional Christian theology would take the same approach. In modern Western thinking there is massive confusion about the words soul and spirit. The word soul can mean an immaterial entity that is separate from but manifest in the body of a human being or indeed an animal, if one believes that there is no real distinction between animals and humans. It is only useful in the context of a dualist picture of humanity. For example, the word soul has meaning if someone believes that at the time of conception an immaterial soul is placed in the body by God, or possibly at some other time. At death, an immaterial soul leaves the body and either joins a resurrected body or has an incorporeal existence. In Hinduism, the spirit or soul seeks release from rebirth, and earthly life is only complete when the soul or animating spirit is released permanently from embodiment. But the real problem for any thinker is how to square all the varied thoughts about the concepts of soul and spirit with what we observe in nature.

In practice, when we use these words we are usually referring to the essence of a person, something that develops over time. If we refer to someone as 'soulless' we are usually suggesting that there is an absence of qualities that we associate with the soul or spirit, such as a loving nature, understanding heart, or wisdom.

As life progresses an entity is built up of many facets. We call that human entity a person. The central question that bothers religious people is the nature of that person. Is the person just a combination of neurones, fibres and synapses or has something more complex emerged that could even have the properties of living on after the body has died? Here we are faced with the ultimate mystery. Brain science does not encourage the concept of an immaterial soul. The well-known neurophysiologist John Eccles considered it was possible and attempted to justify his position, but few working in neuroscience have been encouraged to follow him. Mind and soul are both emergent and may be the same. One could use the word soul to describe the essence of a person but it may be simpler to speak of people who are sometimes referred to as souls. A priest has care of souls but we all realise that this refers to people.

Most of us have never thought it necessary to define any limits of Personhood. People are people. People are in some way special – at least from our point of view. Homo sapiens has attained a unique place on this planet. We can think creatively about our purpose and ultimate destiny, and as far as we know this is unique in the animal world. We are now able to influence the future course of our existence for good or bad.

When does being a person begin? Is an embryo created by in vitro fertilisation a person? If not, what about after implantation, but before there are any recognisable organs? If an embryo is not always a person, then when does it become one? These questions about the nature or definition of a person have become an issue for discussion because of attempts to define personhood for the purposes of medical decision making. I remain unconvinced that this is helpful, but we live in a world where financial pressures can sometimes lead decision makers to seek ways of reducing the burden of prolonged care. It may be appropriate to set the scene with a range of examples that highlight the debate about personhood.

Carol and Jim were unable to have children without recourse to in vitro fertilisation. However, they were very concerned about the implantation of multiple embryos with the attendant risks of multiple pregnancies and the likelihood that embryos would not survive. They decided that they wanted one embryo implanted at a time. They were not experts in ethics but this course seemed right to them. They had no objection to the storage of eggs and sperm because they felt that human life only commences at fertilisation.

Carol and Jim seem to believe that personhood starts at fertilisation, implying that the soul enters the body at that time.

Janice became pregnant by her soldier boyfriend. She was sixteen. He made it clear to her that he did not want a baby and there was no possibility of a permanent relationship. She was very upset. She went to see her general practitioner with her mother. He told her she was a silly girl and would have to take the consequences of her behaviour. There was no possibility of an abortion. Janice did not want to have the baby. It was no more complicated than that. Her mother had another contact and it was arranged for Janice to see a private general practitioner who referred her to hospital where an abortion was carried out on the grounds of her mental distress. She was ten weeks pregnant.

Janice seems to have thought that an embryo was an embryo. She did not believe she was murdering anything or that the early embryo had a unique status.

Baby John had Down's syndrome. Doctors at the hospital informed his parents that he required an abdominal operation to relieve a blocked intestine. They were unhappy about such a procedure. They felt it was better to let John die. The staff did not agree. They took the view that the operation was likely to be successful and that there was no reason why John should not have a reasonable quality of life. He was a person. The matter was taken to court and the parents were overruled.

Baby John was not necessarily thought to be a non-person by his parents, but the hospital staff considered the operation to be perfectly feasible and they were not prepared to see John treated differently to a 'normal' child.

Paul was only eighteen when he sustained a very severe head injury. He was treated in an intensive care unit but survived only in a persistent vegetative state. He was fed artificially. There was no evidence of any awareness. Four years after the original accident the condition remained unchanged and he was cared for in a local hospital. Reluctantly, his parents began to discuss with the staff the possibility of letting Paul die.

Paul's parents remembered him as the 'old Paul'. They thought that his essence had gone. They saw no point in allowing this 'body' to linger. Others would have stated that Paul no longer fulfilled the criteria of personhood.

Sylvia developed progressive dementia when she was around fifty-five years of age. She became so impaired mentally that she did not know who she was or where she was. She did not recognise her husband or children. She could do nothing for herself although she was not paralysed. Eventually she was admitted to a nursing home. The local doctor discussed with her husband the extent to which any illness should be treated.

Sylvia presents a more difficult example of whether someone can value their existence. If her quality of life was very low, was it justified to resort to active intervention should an infection occur?

These brief examples are used to set the background to a debate that developed as to when it is justified, if ever, to make decisions that terminate life or allow death. Perhaps, if someone is not a person, they could be treated in a different way. But the question as to whether something or someone is a person or not is bound to be a value judgement, not a statement of fact subject to verification. That is, unless there is clear consensus about person definitions that leave little or no room for doubt. Beyond these rational arguments the very idea of 'persons' carries with it emotional connotations that reason does not accommodate.

When looking at various objects in nature people may agree in many instances when the word 'person' is appropriate. One would be unlikely to use the word of a stone, a plant, but we may treat animals as if they were people. Although an animal does not use human language, sophisticated communication is apparent between animals of the same species. Humans may form an emotional bond with pets and this increases with time, so that the loss of the pet becomes like a human death. The naming of the animal is an important part of treating it as if it were a person. But it is important to note that we are prepared to kill animals when they are ill enough to have, in our opinion, no quality of life.

In relation to humans the philosopher John Harris raised the question of the nature of persons in his book *The Value of Life – an Introduction to Medical Ethics*. He based his arguments about personhood on whether someone can value their own existence. In his view unless this criterion is present personhood does not exist. There may be potential for it to occur, as in a foetus or a child, but in other situations the criteria for personhood are permanently lost or there is no potential for their development. For one to be able to value one's own life, as far as we know, one must be conscious and aware of self. Presumably one must value the state of life more than death or death more than life. This kind of view of personhood depends on a functioning brain and a kind of brain that can reflect and make decisions; a brain that is far more than a collection of primitive instincts and reflex actions.

We might be able to agree that a being in a persistent vegetative state resulting from a severe head injury is not a person according to this criterion. However, there are difficulties when it comes to looking at boundary criteria. We are unable to make an accurate judgement as to when a child first values its life, nor can we be sure when someone with dementia loses all ability to think and reflect; such issues are not possible to assess with total certainty.

Even if Harris is right in wishing to locate personhood in certain brain conditions it is not always easy to establish their presence or absence.

One of the attractions of a clear definition of personhood is that it seeks to identify what is specific about us. It is assumed that this separates people from animals. Unfortunately, many people fail to reach these exacting criteria at some time in their existence, and the only thing that then separates them from other animals is a difference in species. A severely brain damaged human has less ability and potential than a normal dolphin. There would seem no reason to treat the human differently based on personhood criteria. We do not know whether dolphins can value their lives, but there might be a case for treating them as being of greater moral value than someone in a persistent vegetative state on a simple analysis of brain criteria.

Since the days of *Plato* personhood has been linked with the mind and soul; the body as an integral part of being a person has been despised. In the *Phaedo (64b–65c)* Plato states:

"Then when is it that the soul attains to truth? When it tries to investigate anything with the help of the body it is obviously led astray... Surely the soul can best reflect when it is free from all distractions such as hearing or sight or pain or pleasure of any kind – that is when it ignores the body and becomes as far as possible independent, avoiding all physical contact and associations as much as it can, in its search for reality."

Plato does not equate mind and brain, for him the soul is an immaterial substance that is freed from the body at death. The soul is linked with reason and wisdom and the perfection of humanity, typified by the philosopher. The intellectual pursuit of truth is hindered by the bodily passions. Plato is a dualist and the death of the body, including the brain, presents no problem for him as the soul will survive, eventually to be reborn again, if not in a human then a lower animal. This 'high view' of rationality and intellect at the expense of the body has fostered the view that person's equal mental activity. The body simply does not matter.

Although the body is nothing on its own, the brain is nothing either in isolation. A disembodied brain is not human. Despite the efforts of some theologians to make something of a disembodied eternal life, it is certainly not human. That is not to state it could not exist. The need to postulate some form of eternal body in the Judaeo-Christian understanding of resurrection is to convince us that we survive death in continuity with previous existence.

Human and other animal existence involves the integrated function of the nervous system and the various bodily parts. Mind emerges gradually in the human and all the evidence suggests that it is related to brain size and complexity. Mental activity grows with human maturation. The parts of mental activity that are regarded as related to mind, typically, are rationality, self-awareness, the linking of past present and future events and the sophisticated use of language. It is argued that this is what makes someone a human person rather than a member of the species Homo sapiens. However, is it possible to define the boundary conditions when the human species developed sufficiently to be linked with personhood? Our knowledge of biological evolution would not seem to allow such precision. We do not know when hominids were first able to go beyond their immediate environment and reflect.

Pamela was a young woman with a rare variety of acquired brain damage that exposes some of the difficulties of the concept of personhood and personal identity. At the age of twenty-two, while working as a student nurse, she developed tuberculous meningitis. Despite prompt treatment she developed a profound disorder of memory. She recovered her mobility but was unable to remember much of her past life and could not retain and recall new memory material. For example, if someone performed a painful procedure on her she would have no memory of it a minute or two later despite crying with pain at the time. She had lost the ability to connect the events in her life through memory so that there was no continuity of existence. One could talk with her and she could show emotional responses. She retained the memory for certain tasks so that she could lay the table or do some housework although she could not remember that she had done it. Her life was a series of fragmented events. Based on the following definition of person by John Locke, the English philosopher, she would not meet the criteria:

"A thinking intelligent being that has reason and reflection and can consider itself as that same thinking thing in different times and places; which it does only by that consciousness that is inseparable from it."

In the example of Pamela some features were absent because of the severe disruption of memory, but no one who knew Pamela would wish to deny her the title of person. The features of personhood are those that we as people build up. Most of us have a general idea of what a person is and when asked to produce some analysis will refer to some of the features mentioned. However, we find it much more difficult to state when someone is not a person; that is something we are reluctant to define.

If one considers people with very severe mental impairment, carers with close and prolonged contact with them will be reluctant to deny them the status of person and will be aware of features of their awareness and personality not evident to the casual observer.

I referred in a previous chapter to a middle-aged woman who developed Creutzfeldt-Jakob disease and after a short period passed into a persistent vegetative state. There would be some jaw grinding and the eyes would open. In this situation, most observers considered that the state of death was to be preferred to life. This judgement was not made because it was thought this lady ceased to be a person. The main opinion was that no one should be allowed to lose his or her human dignity in this way. Harris would have argued that she was unable to value her life and it was justified to terminate it and save medical resources.

There was another side to this situation. Joyce's husband wished to keep her alive at all costs. He could not bear the thought of losing his wife. He demanded that the staff do everything possible to keep her alive. He spent much of the day in her company and became aggressive if he considered that his wife was in any way neglected or treated as if she were less than fully conscious. During feeding he criticised the nurses for harming her as he interpreted the jaw grinding and spasm as a distress signal from his wife that she was being hurt. Any rational argument that his wife was no longer a person would have been rejected. He did not accept that his wife was unable to feel or suffer or even think despite her clinical condition. Although his reaction was an extreme one it brings out the point that we do not know what those in persistent vegetative states experience. We cannot know with certainty what is going on and what parts of the brain are dead or alive. Various kinds of brain imaging provide a good deal of evidence nowadays. One can determine the degree of cerebral atrophy, the perfusion of brain parts and their level of activity. But that is only a proxy assessment for what someone might be experiencing. These investigations provide much useful information and are developing all the time, but we cannot state with certainty that bad test results equal a total inability to experience anything, although we may suspect that that is the case.

There is the 'belief' that whatever the appearance of someone the essential self is there, 'locked up' inside the victim of disease. Whether we use the word soul or spirit to describe this is immaterial; it expresses the continuing and unstructured conviction, held by many, that we are more than bodies and brains. Indeed, the word soul rather than refer to a specific entity may be used to refer to that element in human nature that transcends the empirical and material.

Joyce's husband had an experience of what his wife had been over many years. Her personhood for him was made up of a many faceted set of connecting experiences, creating a whole that could not be destroyed by this disease. Her personhood lived independently of the state of her body and brain and continued to do so for him after she was dead. For someone to state that she was no longer a person would appear at best irrelevant, and in the context of his emotional state, obscene. There was an 'eternal' nature about her personhood that could not be reduced to biology or rational statements about her current constitution.

In another situation, the family of Paul took a different view but not because they had any lesser commitment to Paul. They felt the best thing for him was to be allowed to leave this world because he could not live in it. They would suffer whatever happened, but there was nothing more that could be done. They were convinced he had no mental awareness.

One could say that the Paul that had been created over the years had come to an end. There was nothing to be gained by prolonging life. This did not deny that what had been created still existed in the minds of the people who had related to him and continued to be represented by the body; the body remaining a focus for his continued presence in the world.

It would be acceptable to many that Paul die but not by deliberate intent. There would be a difference between nature taking its course and the introduction of lethal material designed to terminate life immediately.

In some cultures, this difference is reflected in the wish to remove the patient from medical care and intervention and return him/her to their home, where death will occur naturally without the confusion generated by modern medical technology.

In human disease and disability, it is important to focus on the body as well as the brain. It seems common sense that we cannot think of personal identity or being a person in terms of brains alone. The original basis of our uniqueness is our genetic constitution. This genetic originality is expressed in our overall make-up; the shape of our bodies, the way we move, our facial appearance, our basic personalities. Our overall identity, including the voice, is heavily influenced by genetics, but we are aware that it is our environment that works with our genetic make-up to complete our uniqueness. A scar of unusual shape and location may serve to distinguish us from others over a span of many years. Our personal identity is not created in the brain alone but in every part of our being. All the nuances of physical behaviour serve to create the totality of an individual human being. The shape and function of the body creates many of the thoughts and dispositions that we experience in our minds. What we are is not susceptible to reductionism. We are the sum of our genetic and environmental interaction.

The concept of personhood that is brain centred is inadequate to encompass persons who have severe neurological disabilities that do not affect higher mental function. When we think of someone we know, their overall appearance matters. We do not reflect on whether they can value their lives. Someone with a severe physical disability is seen by themselves and others as a totality. This applied to the picture that the relatives of Paul and the Husband of Joyce had of their loved ones. Any decisions that were made had no connection with person definitions. They were people whatever happened to them.

Personhood is far too woolly a concept to use as a basis for decision making. One of the problems with ethical debate in health care is a capacity to neglect the emotional and intuitive. Our ethical positions are determined frequently by non-rational elements. For instance, we might take the view that someone on a life support machine is still a person if she is a loved one; we might take a different view if the individual on the machine is a potential donor for a sick relative.

In an article entitled *Do human cells have rights?* Mary Warnock stated: "Personhood is a notoriously difficult and ambiguous concept, and if we can get on without it in this matter, so much the better."

She then quotes an article by John Harris. In this he argued that to ask whether research on human embryos should be permitted and for how long is to ask the question when human life begins to have moral significance. Harris goes on to suggest that this is the same question as when does an embryo become a person? Mary Warnock goes on to state: "That personhood, its possession or non-possession, is as much a question of value as is the question when does human life begin to matter, is hard for people to grasp. And yet it is manifestly the case."

She refers to Locke who pointed out that person questions can only be decided if we come to some collective decision for deciding such issues.

Given that there is an inevitable pluralism about the answers to moral questions, it is confusing to obscure the basic questions by referring to controversial concepts. We can only work towards any consensus by attempting to identify what is at stake in any moral issue that involves the treatment of human beings.

If we start with the basic assumption that all human life matters, we shall want to give a very high priority to treating all forms of human life as ends in themselves. But if this is not tempered in any way by reference to benefits to others we may develop a rigid deontology which will have a far-reaching significance for research on early embryos. This dilemma exposes the problems we have in making difficult decisions. Our emotional reactions result in Emotivism. That means that an ethical framework gives way to 'I approve' or 'I disapprove.' If we conclude that early embryos matter so much that we should not kill them, whatever the gains, it is certainly logical to conclude that killing foetuses and adults is not a good thing either, if the only reason for doing so is the benefit of others, as, for instance, in transplants. However, the debate about what one can do to human embryos and foetuses has one aspect that separates them from other mature forms of life. They do not have a distinctive appearance found in human life from birth onwards. The body has yet to create a distinctive image for us.

The issue of 'mattering' is focussed around brain death criteria. One of the worrying things about these is that the only obvious gain from such definitions is the availability of organs for transplant and the more rapid turnover in intensive care units. It is difficult to sustain the argument that the recommendation of an early demise is based on a morality that the affected individual matters and is being treated as an end rather than a convenience.

It is possible to justify death because the individual matters so much that the state of death is a far better thing than life. One can envisage this possibility in the very severely brain damaged neonate, the individual in a persistent vegetative state or someone with extremely severe pre-senile dementia. The fact that some people can decide for themselves that death is to be preferred to life would support this view.

The way to justify killing early embryos and foetuses, say up to sixteen weeks, is to accord them less moral value. They have no established distinctive individual characteristics. Those who consider that life begins at conception would find this difficult to accept. By this is understood that the process of human existence is part of a continuum and that arguments about appearance have no traction.

The sanctity of life principle is a religious concept but felt by many people who hold no specific religious views. Although couched in dogmatic form by the Church and given the authority of God and Christian tradition, it is externalising what is experienced internally by many. The case against killing embryos and foetuses is often weakened by extremist language, but it remains a matter of judgement as to whether they matter less than maturer forms of human existence.

The overall conclusion that I have reached after a life in clinical practice is that it is necessary to refute the view that persons and personhood can be defined. Following on from that conclusion, I do not consider that the concept has any relevance for moral decision making in health care. The alternative approach is to base decision making on respect for the form of human life involved as an end in itself, and that the degree to which individual life matters is the only basis for decision making. We confer the title of person on individuals by our motives and actions as we encounter them. The Bible does not provide a clear ethical framework. We deceive ourselves if we think it does. One of the major problems we have today is the absence of a clear ethical framework for decision making. The person espousing one religion may agree with the one with no religion for different reasons. If we concentrate on the life of Jesus and regard it as selfless, that is the most important aspect of being a person and having to make decisions about other people. Hard decisions are, by their nature, dilemmas. In every important decision, there is usually a downside. In making the decision we leave behind something important, something that is a loss, whatever our decision may have gained.

Redeemable?

"Israel, put your hope in the Lord, for with the Lord is unfailing
love and with him is full redemption."
Psalm 130.7

It is easy enough to connect with someone who has a serious
physical disease that is genetically determined. We find it much
less easy to cope with the questions raised by serious aberrant
behaviour that may be linked to a person's intrinsic makeup.
There are prolonged debates about the relevance of nature versus
nurture and the importance of each. It is widely accepted that
adverse social circumstances profoundly influence a child's
development. But it is important to come to terms with the fact
that what we are, in terms of personality and behaviour,
connected with our genetic makeup. Social position may be
determined in part by our genes, making it difficult to flourish in
a hierarchical society.

On one side this is an expression of the rich variety of
creation. On the other side, it is highly disturbing to know that
some human beings are far more likely to exhibit violent and
anti-social behaviour. What has this got to say about personal
responsibility? Is such a concept false? Should we accept that
people who have the 'wrong' genes cannot be held responsible
for their conduct, or at the very least, they start with a huge
disadvantage in the task of conforming to standards of reasonable

behaviour. However, not all violent behaviour is the result of social and genetic factors.

Jim had acquired epilepsy. He was thirty-four, unmarried, living with his mother. He did not work regularly. His attacks fell into the category known as complex partial seizures. In the episodes, he would go blank, fiddle with his hands, and sometimes pick up objects. He would be unaware where he was or what he was doing. After most attacks, he had a significant period of automatism when he would be unaware of what was happening and do things without any memory of what they were. In this phase, if interfered with or approached, he could be aggressive.

On one occasion, he was in bed. His mother wanted to do the washing. She made him get up and come down to the kitchen with his dirty clothes. He did not remember what happened. The next thing he knew was that he 'came to' in the kitchen. His mother was lying dead on the floor, strangled. When he realised what had happened he went across to a neighbour and gave himself up.

After a detailed examination of the pattern of his attacks and the circumstances, including a criminal trial for murder at which I was a witness, it was accepted that he killed his mother in a period of post-epileptic automatism. This is a very rare event. Violent behaviour is not an important feature of epilepsy.

In this case Jim was not accountable for his actions. He was a gentle person usually. The event had occurred when the function of his brain was impaired. If we are informed that the person has a disease that impairs brain function, causing abnormal behaviour, we feel more comfortable stating the person is ill and not bad.

In the case of schizophrenia or bipolar affective disorder (manic-depression), we tend to accept that violence directed towards self or others is part of a disease in the same category as any physical disease. There is something chemically wrong with the brain that causes these illnesses. However, not everyone finds it possible to accept that violent behaviour can be due to disease. Some will want to state that the person could have done something else. Violence was not a necessary response to a situation.

The problem becomes more difficult when the disease process is not well defined. There is evidence that within the prison population there is a greater proportion of people with genetic abnormalities pre-disposing towards violence than within the general public. The XYY abnormality and other similar ones, in which there are abnormalities of the sex chromosomes, are examples. It has been suggested also that certain partial chromosome deletions are more prominent amongst prisoners. At the very least this is a disadvantage with respect to the avoidance of violent behaviour. Impulse control is a complex subject and is affected by many factors that include acquired brain damage, drugs, cultural norms and genetic constitution.

Research has identified that in the group of people specifically defined as psychopaths, there is an abnormality in brain function. There is a tendency to apply the label 'psychopath' to anyone exhibiting antisocial behaviour but the definition is more specific. A psychopath exhibits antisocial behaviour of a sexual, violent or power/money oriented nature and exhibits no remorse. The behaviour seems to be goal related. Volumetric studies of the amygdaloid nucleus in such subjects have shown reduced volume and responsiveness. This part of the brain is important in emotional responses. Are such people bad or ill? Are they accountable? The question whether such conditions are treatable is an open one.

The basic problem for any simplistic theology of human accountability is that some people are so disadvantaged that their room for freedom of choice, if it exists at all, is seriously undermined. What society tends to do is judge them, marginalise them and exacerbate the distortion. People who have behavioural problems arising from genetic defects presumably require the optimum resources and facilities to help them. The alternative view is that no intervention will make a difference.

One theological challenge is how people with serious behavioural problems fit in to the idea that all humanity is created in the image of God. I doubt if there is a satisfactory response to this question. It is very important to challenge cosy theological views of God and the world. One can attempt an explanation but for many there will be no answer.

There have been other references to the risks of creation, the capacity for things to go wrong during the exploration of creative potential. What is the purpose of creation? We impose our own ideas of what that might be but most people consider that meaning stems from the kind of life we construct through our engagement with the world. But the nature of creation, as we currently understand it, is bound to be associated in some instances with genetic disadvantage that prevents peaceful interaction and ethical conduct. Perhaps there is potential for some of this to be controlled or even treated in the future. However, genetic manipulation has significant ethical challenges. We may be happy to support eliminating genes that cause serious physical diseases; but if we attempt to alter the brain in any way through manipulating genes we become much more concerned. Increasing intelligence may concern us. Do we want to alter people's personalities? If we are able to change aspects of human constitution we become like gods. All this presupposes that we do have some ability to make choices and that our freedom is not illusory.

In theological language one can express this as becoming god-like, workers with or against God. As creation is located in space-time this implies that if we want to think about it in a linear way, humans and any species that succeeds us, are essential parts of making our world a better place. We may not be working with a god who has got it all sorted on his/her own. There is always the possibility that creation could end in disaster and God would not be able to prevent it. This kind of thinking about God is implicit in some of the ideas of process theology that postulates that God develops along with creation.

For God and sentient beings 'becoming' is a painful process; failure is a possibility. One Christian response is that there is no other way of creating anything.

Psychopaths present a problem to theologians. Psychopathy is not currently regarded by some as a mental illness. The cause is ill understood, but the evidence is that genetic factors are relevant. As has been stated Psychopaths are relatively amoral. They may not show genuine remorse for their actions, which implies there is a high probability of anti-social acts being repeated.

One theological challenge of psychopathy is whether it represents a condition that cannot be redeemed. Can a psychopath genuinely repent and change? At the heart of Christianity is the message that we should repent of our sin, our alienation from God and seek to lead a new life. Is the existence of people who cannot do this fatal to Christianity?

One can argue that there is an ability to change and the negative view of the psychopath is fundamentally flawed. But it seems much easier for some people to live a Christian life than others. I do not refer to a propensity to enjoy church going or giving intellectual assent to doctrinal propositions that lead to the 'fruits of the spirit.' One could become involved in arguments about election and pre-destination but these simply do not appeal to me at all.

Human diversity is a rich treasure house but there does seem to be a real problem when it comes to people fitting readily into a fixed religious structure. We do not all have the same capacity for belief or faith. Our differing temperaments and cultures indicate that uniformity of worship is completely unrealistic. Any great religion requires sufficient flexibility to encompass all peoples. How can any 'true religion' exclude people who are born with major disadvantages? For a variety of reasons, it is evident that the human capacity for choice is severely restricted, probably for us all, but certainly for those born into poverty, people with severe physical and mental impairment and those people unfortunate enough to have personalities that cripple their positive engagement in the world.

Words Fail me

"People often complain that music is too ambiguous, that what they should think when they hear it is so unclear, whereas everyone understands words. With me, it is exactly the opposite, and not only with regard to an entire speech but also with individual words."
Felix Mendelssohn

All our attempts to use words are fraught with problems. We struggle to give meaning to our utterances and for the most part it is very unsatisfactory. I was brought up in a religious tradition that was very wordy and very dogmatic. The passage of time and my experiences as a neurologist and someone on a spiritual journey has left me profoundly dissatisfied with most words. Wittgenstein had a student and friend, Maurice O'C Drury, who considered that the philosopher recognised that words said very little about much that is important in life, leaving room for the mystical.

I recognise in the work of the poet an attempt to create a picture that transcends the actual words on the page. Without poetry, we lack one of the gateways to deeper meaning. But poetry is not the only gateway. Art and music are our aids as well.

The struggle of the poet or author to reveal that which lies beneath the events, the narratives of life, is the same struggle for the musician and the artist. The struggle is never over, always incomplete.

Words are symbols that we use to communicate within ourselves and with each other. They are not absolute entities but tools. We give objects in the outside world names: we name the parts of our bodies and those of other creatures. We use words to express ideas, thoughts, and feelings. We use different languages in different cultures. We use words to record our knowledge. The problem is that some people cannot understand language and they may have complete inability to express themselves. These problems may not be total, but they expose for us all the vulnerability at the heart of language. The deaf person can communicate through manual symbols and lip reading, but someone with the medical condition of aphasia has damage to the brain that impairs the capacity to understand and express language. The details of the deficits vary with the individual and the site of brain damage.

Peggy was sixty-five. She was an active married lady without disability and fully engaged in her local community. One evening her husband noticed that she was dribbling fluid from the right corner of her mouth and when he spoke to her to ask how she was there was no reply. Subsequently, Peggy was diagnosed as having sustained a stroke. This had involved the language areas of her brain. After several days she began to speak but it was gibberish to the ordinary listener. There were fragments of words, largely disconnected from any meaningful content. Peggy could not understand what was said to her and was unable to respond to simple commands on a consistent basis. She was unaware that people could not understand what she was saying and became frustrated and depressed. The weakness of the right face resolved and there was no major weakness of the right arm or leg.

Sadly, the language problem did not resolve despite intensive speech and language assessment and therapy. Peggy lived in an isolated world, unable to communicate as she used to. Her social roles disappeared and she was dependent on her husband. Sometimes it was possible to hear meaningful fragments when she was not tired and in the more familiar automatic areas of language. Peggy could no longer read.

We take words for granted in our relationship to the world. They can be effective tools in allowing us to be independent. But language is fragile. It is easily lost.

We may reflect that if language and human thought can reveal ultimate things to us we are using an imperfect tool. Although the development of language has made us apparently successful as a species in developing sophisticated communication and knowledge, there are serious limits to what it can contribute about ultimate mysteries.

If we are inclined to a religious interpretation of the world, believing in an ultimate reality beyond our knowledge and apprehension, language cannot do justice to our religious experiences. Religious or theological language is an imprecise vehicle. It is very easy to slip into the error of assuming that religious or doctrinal statements have the same status as something we deem to be verifiable. The philosophy of Logical Positivism has caused huge problems. Although discredited, it continues to influence the way people think about religious truth. Analytical philosophy has dominated Anglo-American studies until recently. The emphasis on taking apart the constituents of language and ignoring the broader scope of continental philosophy has done nothing to enable the poetic and artistic aspects of communication. The Bible is held up by many as a series of statements that can be treated as simple matters of fact. But the heart of any religion is the experience of the Divine, which by its nature cannot be adequately expressed. Christianity, by emphasising the presence of God in the person of Jesus, can err in attempting to reduce the mystery of God to manageable form. Making 'factual' statements about Jesus is seen as quite legitimate, although in reality they lure us in to overconfidence that we have all the answers or the only answer in Jesus.

Jesus is 'Son of Mary, Son of David, Son of Man, Son of God, born of the Holy Spirit, the Lamb of God, the Christ and The Incarnate Word. These rich expressions are part of our religious heritage. Many of them are ways of expressing the importance of Jesus in our religious experience. They attempt to point to a reality beyond the words. But the words are words. They are often said to be 'inspired'. This is an attempt to give them superior status. But in the end, they are mere words and are the product of the human mind. Of course, it is comforting to imagine that God just speaks words of truth through human mouthpieces. It is surely better to recognise that words are human tools and nothing more. They do give expression to our religious experiences but we are reducing God if we give them a status beyond what they can do for us.

If we state that Jesus is the son of Mary, this could be true to the extent that a woman called Mary gave birth to a child called Jesus in the usual way. In our language we would use the word son to describe this filial relationship. If we state that Jesus is the Son of God we enter different territory. God is not human; He/She is beyond space and time, has no gender, cannot be described, and does not give birth in the human sense of that phrase. The words are used by Christians to describe the importance of Jesus in the Christian religion. Son is an indicator of his closeness to God. It cannot describe a physical relationship. The language is metaphorical. Other words and phrases are used to explore this closeness. God is described as incarnate in Jesus. God dwells in Jesus. Jesus becomes God as the second person of the Trinity. Yet he is a man. We assume he was a historical person. We search for words to describe his religious importance. At one extreme we come to the point when it is stated that Jesus is 'God's only Son'. We have then reached a point when the religion is placing very clear demarcation lines. The experience of some people compels them to make this exclusive statement as a response to their experience. They cannot believe that God could be incarnate other than in Jesus.

Other faiths have looked at religious experience in a different way. They have used words that have a different emphasis. Both Judaism and Islam have recognised the spiritual importance of certain individuals; the word prophet is used to describe many of them. None has the status of God. There is one God. Mohammed, Moses, and others are not understood as incarnations of God in the same way as Jesus in Christianity. Language is less 'stressed' in the other religions of the Book. Hinduism is rich in metaphor and differs from Christianity because the words and stories do not carry the same historical burden. The claim that Christianity is a historical religion may appear to make the use of language easier but this is illusory. The development of Christian doctrine has caused great problems because of the inadequacy of words to express convictions. One could argue that the development of doctrine has reduced Christianity rather than enhancing it. It has created a false certitude.

In Hinduism words about the nature of the 'One' or the source of all being are more restricted, despite the vast Vedic literature. The word Brahman is used to describe the Godhead and Atman that divine spark within each creation. The word OM made up of the sounds AUM is the all in all.

"OM, the eternal word is all. What was, what is, and what shall be, and what is beyond is in eternity; all is OM."

Mandukya Upanishad

Hinduism is a mythological, incarnational religion. That may appear a contradiction. However, figures such as Krishna and Rama fulfil a similar role to Jesus. How much would it matter if Jesus was not an historical person? Would his 'story' have the same impact? It may be assumed that Krishna was not historical but some people disagree. It does not matter. The existence of a Kuru kingdom is widely accepted in Indian history. Krishna may have been the preeminent statesman and philosopher of the time. He was later identified as an avatar of Vishnu. In a similar sense Rama may have existed as a major Aryan chieftain who led an expedition to Sri Lanka. Since Buddha is considered as a historical figure and an avatar of Vishnu so why not Krishna and Rama? Teachings in the Bhagavad Gita and Ramayana have historical impact regardless of the historicity of the protagonists. The sacred literature contains many words but no structured orthodox dogma. The Vedic scriptures are poetic structures originating over vast tracts of time. The figures of Brahma, Vishnu and Shiva symbolise aspects of existence; creation, sustaining and destruction. Much is left unsaid.

When we try to use words to attempt to express profound spiritual insights there may be coherence of the words used. This is unsurprising. However, in the varying traditions we find differences in the use of poetic language. If one compares the following two examples from the Rig Veda and Genesis there is a difference in the use of imagery. The account in Genesis does not evoke the same sense of mystery. It is accepted that translation does affect the impact of any words. Nuances are lost.

"There was not then what is or what is not. There was no sky, and no heavens beyond the sky... There was neither death nor immortality then. No signs were there of night or day. The ONE was breathing by its own power, in deep peace. Only the ONE was; there was nothing beyond... and in the ONE arose Love. Love the first seed of soul."

Rig Veda X. 129

"In the beginning God created the heavens and the earth. Now the earth was formless and empty, darkness was over the surface of the deep, and the Spirit of God was hovering over the waters."

Genesis 1.1-2

Our own religious traditions, deeply embedded in our cultures, may be true or right for us; but it is important that we recognise the limitations of all religious structures, all religious words. It is appropriate to worship God from within one's own world. It is very difficult to worship, using different sacred literature from another tradition. Where a religion has a rich oral and written history it is not the norm to move from one religion to another. All concepts dependant on language are frail vehicles of the ultimate: God, Om, Allah, Yahweh.

The younger generation in the West find Christians have been inculcated with empiricism. This makes it difficult for them to engage with ancient dogma presented as the core of their cultural inheritance. However, they retain a sense of mystery, the unknown, the extraordinary nature of the natural world. Many feel connected with the environment and see themselves as different rather than 'special'. Concepts separating humans from animals are a cause for concern. Language that gives humans souls and not animals is rejected. Speciesism concerns them. Thus the 'image of God' metaphor troubles them. Peter Singer, the Australian philosopher considers Speciesism is an attitude of bias against a being because of the species to which it belongs. Humans show speciesism when they give less weight to the interests of nonhuman animals than they give to the similar interests of human beings. The reason for mentioning this is that religious words and language that separate humans from the natural world may hamper a recognition of our essential unity with everything. Although the 19th century reaction to *Evolution by Natural Selection* appears to have been resolved in main stream Christianity, closer inspection raises doubts that human evolution from 'simpler' life forms has fully entered theological discourse.

Future religious language may need to embody these renewed understandings. Renewed, because our early ancestors understood their connection to the natural word better than we do. Many wish to worship and explore spiritually, but Christianity is rapidly losing touch with people. This is the fault of the Church and the barren nature of much theological discourse and language. The broad Church will eventually be forced in to a reappraisal of how religious language incorporates our essential unity with everything else in nature rather than our 'specialness'. Some progress has been made, but much more creative thinking is required. Eastern religions have always recognised this unity.

Looser knit religions can retain younger generations. At a recent Bengali wedding, it was clear that the rituals and ancient Sanskrit words were an integral part of family tradition. The young people did not take these things literally but they acknowledged the collective spiritual wisdom and insight of their culture that lay beyond words or concepts.

Returning to a medical practitioner's concerns about language, one thing is self-evident. Many members of the human race are unable to use language to explore ultimate reality. My own understanding has become less dependent on words despite spending a lifetime using them. Sometimes, when I look at words on a page my mind freezes; the words 'stare' at me. They have no meaning. My solution is to look at something in the world around me; the wordless environment of nature or even urban sprawl. When I hear words they sometimes inspire me but mostly confuse me. Somehow. I am left dissatisfied. They fail to capture the ineffable. Some mornings, I sit in my wheelchair after a shower and gaze through the window. The view is nothing special but on occasion it takes me beyond myself to a reassuring presence that requires no language. Any truth for the religious person must lie beyond words however imaginatively we use them to touch the eternal, beyond our senses.

Encounter and Expectation

"I never promised you a rose garden."
The title of a novel by Hannah Green

The starting point was usually a letter. The letter arrived at the hospital addressed to the consultant, in this case a neurologist. The letter was about a person. The length and content would vary depending on the referring general practitioner and the reason for referral. In some cases, the diagnosis was already made and the letter requested advice on management of symptoms or the reduction of disability. Many letters recorded the medical history, requesting advice about diagnosis and treatment. Sometimes the purpose of the consultation was to reassure someone.

An appointment was offered. The individual along with others designated for a clinic attended the outpatients department. Each new encounter was allocated twenty to thirty minutes. Despite these limitations clinics usually overran. The unwritten rule was that no consultation should be aborted because of time restrictions. The demand for services was such that that these sessions would tax the mental and emotional resources of the clinic staff. Every session was conducted against the background awareness of the length of the waiting list and the need to be 'efficient.'

After the consultant had read the letter the patient was invited to enter the consulting room. The challenge was to make contact, enable that person to describe their problems, elicit the relevant background and clarify symptom details, make a physical examination, come to some conclusions and talk with the person. Arrange, if necessary, the appropriate investigations. Each contact was a kind of adventure, containing risk, the outcome uncertain. This was the same for everyone in the room. Much of the time it was not possible to predict what these face to face contacts would lead to. How the story would be told and what the interpretation would be was an unknown. Although the background to the medical role was science, each episode was unique, with a mysterious, even sacred quality. Much of the time for the neurologist there was a sense of inadequacy, not because of lack of knowledge, but because of the need to enter a life, make a connection. Was what presented the real issue? Or was there some deeper dis-ease beneath the surface? How could one achieve anything in twenty minutes?

We spend our lives involved in encounters. The shape of our expectations may be influenced by our fiduciary framework. Belief in the active intervention of God in our personal world may influence us unhealthily; make it difficult to accept adverse findings and promote selfishness in our search for salvation. The novel by Hannah Green referred to is partly autobiographical. A girl with schizophrenia struggles with her disease and the consequences and is helped by a therapist to deal with her reality rather than torment herself with false expectations. What we expect varies. Even for the physician there can be no uniform pattern. The most mundane one is to get through the clinic in time and with no major mishaps, no confrontations, and no angst.

There could be the expectation of encountering an unusual clinical situation that taxed the intellect, stimulated the interest of a tired mind.

For the person attending the clinic the variation in expectations would be much wider. Many would come seeking reassurance, a harmless diagnosis, nothing too serious. Living with the symptoms would be easy after reassurance. Others knew the diagnosis but sought help and support in living with incurable disease. They needed advice about aids, symptom management, and a talk about the future. Some had little insight into their symptoms, they were suffering from inner turmoil, mental anguish, and a need for healing that did not fit a simple medical model.

In some instances, the patient could not understand why they had fallen victim to disease. They associated an upright life with health and prosperity. They felt let down.

The doctor would be aware that some of those attending had no interest in him. They came for some answers. He was not a person but a means of providing information, diagnosis, and cures. He would be judged on his performance. In some instances, if he was unable to provide the cure required he was rejected, along with the diagnosis.

Sometimes the neurologist thought of himself as an interpreter of dreams. An experience reminded him of Joseph. In the book of Genesis, the Pharaoh imprisoned Joseph for a time. He was given responsibility over the other prisoners. Two people imprisoned came to him with dreams for interpretation. One, the king's cupbearer received an encouraging interpretation and was rapidly restored; the other, the baker was less fortunate and was executed. There were no apparent reasons for these random events.

Two people, known to each other, attended the same clinic. They were concerned about unusual symptoms.

The first gave his account of tingling and numbness in the hands and feet that had progressed. The examination revealed physical signs that raised the possibility of the diagnosis of vitamin B12 deficiency that can cause a disease known as sub-acute degeneration of the spinal cord. The person, James, was very worried that he had an incurable disease. Investigations confirmed vitamin B12 deficiency and with lifelong injections of vitamin B12 the symptoms and signs regressed and eventually resolved completely. James moved on and lived a normal fulfilled life in retirement.

His close friend Colin came with a story of flickering of his muscles and weakness in one leg. Despite the localised nature of the weakness, examination suggested widespread abnormalities due to a condition known as motor neurone disease.

There is no cure and most people die within five years of the onset with progressive widespread paralysis. The muscles for swallowing and speech are frequently involved.

Investigations confirmed this diagnosis. It was not possible to give Colin good news. His story was very different to that of James. The disease progressed inexorably. He appeared to face it with calm acceptance. There was no happy retirement and he died within three years of the onset.

The issues that underlie these encounters have caused me to reflect on the core elements that make them worthwhile. Consultations are so numerous for the average doctor that it is easy to be swamped by the volume of experience and be unable to reflect adequately on it. I have spent plenty of time on both sides of the consultation process and this has enabled me to evaluate what seems to be important.

Apart from clinical ability and scientific knowledge. the aspect that strikes me most forcibly from both sides is the ability to listen.

The willingness and ability to listen is of great spiritual significance. At the heart of a Christian understanding of God is that he knows us and listens to us. For me the collect of purity summarises this:

"Almighty God to whom all hearts are open, all desires known, and from whom no secrets are hidden: cleanse the thoughts of our hearts by the inspiration of your Holy Spirit that we may perfectly love you and worthily magnify your holy name; through Jesus Christ, our Lord."

Listening is about being open and about love. It is meant to be reciprocal. On many occasions, I have failed to listen or be listened to. As a doctor in a busy clinic I have 'switched off' when people with severe problems related to disability are describing their needs. Sometimes this has been because I did not know what to do about them. Sometimes it was weariness, inability to concentrate or disinterest. One would make automatic responses and grunt or say 'yes' and 'no' at the appropriate times.

As a patient, I have been only too aware that I was not being heard. The impact on me was usually to make me feel a burden and to be very selective about what I said so that the catalogue was not too extensive. There is merit in this. It is better to concentrate on the most active problems if you can. However, the lay person cannot be expected to be able to filter them in the same way as a medically qualified patient. But it did make me angry if

I was not heard; it made me reluctant to go again. It is not that people expect easy answers necessarily. They hope for patience and understanding and a sharing. That is therapeutic in itself. Without listening one is not at the beginning of a real encounter.

It is reasonable to suggest that in some areas of medicine it may be possible to function with skill and yet be a poor listener and communicator. Someone might suggest that they would prefer to have their hip replaced by a good surgeon even if he is rude and does not listen. There is then a minimal encounter. It may work if the problem is straightforward but it is a matter of technical ability and knowledge divorced from caring.

What should one expect from our health care encounters? We have an over-stressed under-resourced Health Service. Staff are increasingly criticised publicly and are often demoralised. They may feel that they are at the sharp end of consumer demand rather than in a relationship of mutual trust where each party recognises the others humanity and limitation. Dedication and commitment may become soured and worn down. The patient should certainly expect clinical knowledge and skill, politeness and a caring attitude. In return the staff has reason to anticipate that there is mutuality in the encounter and it is not merely a matter of laying a problem at someone else's feet and expecting an instant solution.

False expectation is a serious problem. It is unfortunate that Health Service staff can become the substitute for a good friend, an understanding clergy-person, and the family. It is common for emotional and relationship problems to be expressed in physical symptoms with the expectation that they have some ready panacea in a visit to the doctor. Surgeries and hospitals are clogged up with people who do not need to be there, who do not require the medical model to solve their ills, or who have minor problems that can be dealt with at home by themselves. There is an obsession with 'health', but it is divorced by many from spiritual wellbeing.

At the core of any encounter should be the realisation that 'cure' is not the only possible outcome. It has become fashionable to view medicine as a series of technological breakthroughs that allow successful treatment of an ever-increasing number of disorders. This truth is partial. There are large numbers of people of all ages with 'incurable disease'. Many of these are diseases of the nervous system. Whatever the future may hold this is present reality.

In this situation the encounter may take place over years. The visits are a listening and sharing experience. There is the possibility of solving some problems together, of making a difference to quality of life, but there is no expectation of cure. The parties both know that this is not in the nature of things. Over the years the nurse, doctor or any other member of the caring professions, is affected by the relationship.

Jim came to see me with his parents over many years until I retired. He had severe cerebral palsy. Apart from paralysis in all limbs his body was wracked by frequent involuntary torsion movements that affected his neck, tongue, trunk and limbs.

He was unable to speak. It was necessary to feed Jim with great care because swallowing was impaired severely. He was liable to recurrent chest infections.

Jim was seated in a specially constructed frame for his wheelchair but even with many trials at the seating clinic the posture of his body was grossly distorted.

Within this broken body was a lively intelligence with a great sense of humour. Although Jim could not speak himself, with the assistance of a special communication aid he could choose short sentences that spoke for him with an American accent.

Over the years there were many crises to overcome but Jim could expand his surroundings with his own group of young carers. He became established in an extension of the family home.

The encounter with him was life enhancing for me. Jim symbolised the beauty of the human spirit that transcends a broken body. It has helped me to understand that God is not a god of physical perfection, of easy answers, but a god present in broken people. Perfection in the spiritual sense is nothing to do with how we look, how we think, how we function physically. Once we have encountered those who are truly alive despite grave disadvantages we are humbled, made to reflect on our own selfishness and petty concerns. People like Jim are constant reminders to us that our own lives mean little if divorced from the broken, the marred, and the marginalised.

Blame and Stress

"I did not hide my face from mocking and spitting.
Because the Sovereign Lord helps me, I will not be disgraced.
Therefore have I set my face like flint, and I know I will not be
put to shame."
Isaiah 50.6–7

It is easier to give examples of stress than define it. Like most things some level of mental stress is normal and healthy. It is part of life. To expect a life free of it is completely unrealistic. Stress is not an absolute; coping capacities vary. We can make our own stress through our own decisions and behaviour. There is some evidence that strong religious belief may reduce anxiety, providing the type of belief is not dominated by guilt and anxiety about divine judgement. A small part of the brain, the anterior cingulate gyrus, becomes stimulated when someone is anxious and is less activated in committed believers. However, we may find ourselves in situations that are chronically stressful and the resolution of the problems largely beyond our control. Those who claim that they are never stressed may not have engaged with life. They have done or risked nothing. TS Eliot, described in his poem *The Hollow Men* those unengaged people, straw stuffed, shadowy figures. He was influenced by Dante. In the *Divine Comedy* there are those who stand at the entrance to Hell or the Inferno. They cannot enter because they have done nothing. One is reminded of the servant given one talent. He buried it. There was no engagement in life. For those of us who attempt to live purposefully, blame culture enhances stress. We blame each other for the decisions that did not work out. Society tends to focus blame on individuals for adverse events. This is seen to provide 'closure'.

The professions of medicine and nursing are inherently stressful because of the exposure of ordinary individuals to many people with serious disease, in vulnerable states, seeking help. Within the medical profession there has been increasing realisation that stress management is important. Medical staff easily become isolated. The doctor has traditionally been the accountable figure in health care decisions. Doctors have not had a good record of working in teams, amongst themselves or with other professional groups.

The accustomed manner of ensuring accountability in hospital medicine is to register the patient with a particular consultant for any episode. Although this has many advantages, it does encourage isolationism within clinical practice, particularly if the relevant doctor has an innate difficulty in seeking advice. It is now accepted that there has been great reluctance for clinicians to show formal concern about their immediate colleagues' performance. This has led to several well-publicised cases of alleged or proven clinical incompetence. The secondary effect of these events has been to create a climate of 'doctor bashing'. A culture of blame is now endemic. The medical profession is under great stress. Morale in hospitals is probably at an all-time low level. There is now serious concern that future generations will have no desire to practise medicine in a climate of hostility and over-regulation. There is a very

179

narrow line between proper accountability and stifling over-regulation that appears to have been crossed. Some of this is the fault of the profession that has over-reacted to individual crises, but the media, public and government must take responsibility. The use of unbalanced emotive language has created a culture that has severely damaged considered opinion and thoughtful strategy.

The public rightly wants to be able to place their trust in doctors but at the same time the demanding and stressful aspects of medical practice require recognition. Doctors are beginning to perceive themselves as 'monitored for error' in a way that undermines the nature of the profession. There is serious risk of eroding any idea of medicine as a vocation. Unless some correctives are applied there is a real possibility that it will be quite impossible to pursue a vocation within such a stifling environment. Instead of achieving the goal of better quality care for all, those driving the 'doctor bashing' culture may create a situation that is dominated by severe staff shortages, reduced availability and standards of medical care, and the ultimate total disintegration of health care in the United Kingdom. This may appear alarmist but it would be wise to take the situation very seriously.

One of the greatest threats to sensible arrangements for medical accountability and a fair system for monitoring performance is the 'knee jerk' reaction to specific events that results in ill-thought-out general and sweeping changes. Public expectation has understandably increased concerning medical care, but the realities of the pressures on all health care staff have not been fully appreciated. It is very difficult indeed for people to work in an environment dominated by criticism rather than affirmation, by lack of human resources, and in some instances by inadequate equipment.

The starting point ought to be that staff have the patient's interest at heart and are committed and skilled professionals. If one accepts this premise, over regulation of caring professions could result in reduced standards not higher ones. Unfortunately, this fear is gradually being realised. There is a crisis in the recruitment and retention of doctors and nurses. Despite assurances that more doctors and nurses will be in post, the United Kingdom is becoming more dependent on procuring staff from other countries to prop up the Health Service. Because of the cultural aspects of good health care, it is unwise to assume that increased numbers, regardless of origin, will equate with better health care.

Acceptance of each other is a core feature of the Christian gospel. We believe that God accepts us as we are, but calls us to a life of seeking to transcend our basic selfishness and learn how to serve others. Jesus has become our model for this.

This acceptance requires mutual trust between people; we cannot accept each other without exercising this. Suspicion, fear and blame are inimical to trust. What has happened in recent years is that the level of complaints against doctors has increased substantially, but there is no good evidence that the standards of the profession are lower. New technology and treatments bring different ways of doing things. Medical knowledge has increased dramatically and will continue to do so. But changes in knowledge are not the real issue. What is important is the erosion of trust.

It is vital not to equate trust with that well-worn phrase, 'you know best doctor'. There is no reason at all why there should not be mutual sharing of information, including the difficulties that may beset any clinical situation.. All staff need to feel comfortable about seeking advice and being able to ask their colleagues freely for help. It is not a sign of failure to ask for a second opinion.

What has gone wrong with the trusted doctor-patient relationship? In many instances, nothing at all. However, the profession has been slow to adapt to a greater desire on the part of the majority for full explanations and involvement in all decisions. Secrecy has been a failing in some doctors and secrecy is the enemy of trust. The Christian gospel is quite clear that we should not be afraid of the truth. 'It will set us free'. I find some connection between fear of openness within health care and that within the church. It is vital that all Christians share doubts and difficulties without fear of censure and rejection.

Many people have developed quite unrealistic expectations about health. As a society, we are unhealthily involved in contemplating our own individual wellbeing. Health has become one of the modern gods that we worship and there is a tendency to be angry and complain when our goals are not realised. This may lead to stress amongst those who seek to satisfy unreasonable demands. Sometimes people move between many health care workers until they are satisfied or blame everyone for their failure to have their needs met. There are numerous examples in health care of individual selfishness in securing resources for our own wellbeing at the expense of others. Those who need the most help are often those who do not receive it.

The Christian gospel is radical. Although some perceive it to be largely about individual salvation, it is difficult to envisage how individual salvation can have any meaning at all when others suffer. The cults of individualism, blame and complaint are closely linked.

Many complaints, after investigation, are totally unjustified. They result in a waste of time and resources. Some complaints are. Some people never complain but should do so. It is quite impossible to obtain a clear picture of how to regulate a profession based on complaints.

It is completely unrealistic to expect to develop a system that results in perfect clinical practice. We will all make mistakes. What is important in medicine and nursing is to hold on to the possibility that people will choose these professions through a sense of vocation. If these elements are there we are more likely to have carers who are motivated to serve. They will want to be as good at their jobs as possible. That is the essence of vocation. However, they will feel threatened and unaccepted by restrictive monitoring. Society needs to allow the professions the time and space for development and training and be positive not negative about the people it turns to for health problems.

We sometimes hear a politician utter the words: 'This must never happen again'. In the context of medicine, this may mean that an adverse event, or series of events, requires radical change in monitoring structures to prevent its recurrence. Detailed examination of such episodes can reveal that the factors operative in any adverse situation are more complex than is honestly admitted or realised, and the prescribed solution over-elaborate or simplistic; too often a reaction to pressure groups or public outcry insufficiently informed.

After a career in clinical medicine physical disability necessitated a change of direction and the neurologist accepted a part time post as medical director of a newly formed NHS Trust alongside a modest amount of clinical work. This was a major change of direction dictated by physical limitation. Although the neurologist was respected by his colleagues and encouraged to take on the role, the concept of medical director was not well defined at that time. However, it seemed appropriate to appoint a senior member of the profession with extensive committee experience.

After about a year the local press leaked information about a consultant at the hospital that was very unfavourable to that person. Although the newly appointed medical director was unaware of any adverse background, it transpired that the doctor's senior colleague, the chairman of the Trust and director of human resources, were acquainted with the information leaked. The information centered on the fact that prior to taking up a consultant post in the United Kingdom the doctor had been struck off the medical register in another country for clinical malpractice. Information was also made available that local police had cautioned the same doctor about his conduct in a public lavatory.

This information entered the public domain in 1993, but the doctor had apparently been successfully employed as a consultant in the NHS since early 1985. His clinical colleagues had not complained about his work. He was respected in the region, had been elected to the fellowship of the relevant Royal College and was a member of several important local and regional committees.

His contract of employment had been held until 1992 by the local regional health authorities until NHS reorganisation resulted in their abolition and the creation of local NHS Trusts. It became clear that he had been selected through the usual interview process with outside assessors and appropriate references.

It transpired that the regional health authority had learned of the trouble in another country sometime after the appointment in 1985. The General Medical Council was informed and this would have happened anyway, as a matter of routine, by the overseas regulatory authority. The General Medical Council could have investigated the matter, but it would have required a detailed hearing with overseas witnesses. At the time, they considered it beyond their jurisdiction. A private investigation by the health authority that included sending information concerning the charges to a senior member of the profession saw no cause for revoking the appointment, for special monitoring, or any other measures.

The local Trust decided to carry out an investigation as to the facts of the consultant's practice in the UK in 1993. The Trust records contained no abnormal body of complaints against the doctor and his work. Consultation with his immediate past and present colleagues provided a picture of clinical competence. There were no substantive complaints from general practitioners. The local community health council had no record of complaint. Clinical colleagues in the hospital were angry that the consultant should be bothered in this way. They supported him fully.

The enquiry could find no factual evidence that the consultant had performed inadequately in the UK, and it was considered that the previous private enquiry of the regional authority and the decision of the GMC were matters that could not be reopened.

The consultant continued working, albeit with arrangements in place that made it possible for people disturbed by the news leaks to be treated by other doctors. As it happened, there was no significant change in referral patterns. However, the consultant was asked to take a lower profile and much of his committee work diminished.

It became clear that he was becoming demotivated and less interested in his work.

His immediate clinical colleagues became less supportive. The Chief Executive of the Trust considered it appropriate to look at the issue again, and on this occasion the Trust produced some charges relating to relatively minor issues, unconnected with clinical expertise. The medical director had no role in preparing these charges, which were vigorously rebutted by the consultant. The British Medical Association, representing him, considered them to be 'trumped up.'

The Medical Director was asked to chair the hearing and prior to this the consultant was suspended by the director of human resources. In the National Health Service suspension is a neutral act and does not imply guilt of any charges.

On the day of the hearing the consultant attended with his legal team and announced that he no longer wished to work for the Trust and would take no part in the hearing. He stated that he would agree to negotiations to secure an agreement for him to leave the Trust.

Subsequently, the director of human resources, with legal input from both sides, brokered an agreement that included the lifting of the suspension and all charges, and a period of paid sabbatical leave for one year and an employer's reference. The content of the reference had to be agreed by the two parties. The medical director was to sign the reference on behalf of the Trust.

The agreement was eventually signed. The consultant was offered a locum appointment in another town, and the medical director signed a brief reference confirming that the doctor had performed satisfactorily in his ten years with the hospital and was now looking for a change of direction. The matters already looked at by the GMC and regional health authority were not referred to, nor was the suspension as no allegations had been proven, and no suspension existed following the cessation of charges.

Subsequently, the consultant had difficulties at the locum appointment. Someone ill disposed towards him leaked the original news of his problems outside the UK, and the episode in the public lavatory. His appointment was terminated, but he went on to obtain locum appointments at other hospitals, utilising other referees, and worked also at a private clinic. The Trust provided no further references.

However, approximately three years after his departure from the Trust the consultant became the subject of adverse publicity about his work in the United Kingdom despite the previous opinions expressed about his clinical competence. Some former patients established a group complaining about their treatment. A great deal of publicity ensued leading to an enquiry by the General Medical Council, who found the consultant guilty of serious professional misconduct and removed his name from the medical register.

A great deal of anger was directed towards the Trust where he worked originally. Managers were blamed for employing the doctor and for giving him a reference on his departure that was described as 'glowing'. The fact that they had not employed him originally, and the absence of complaints at an earlier stage, were glossed over. An independent review of his clinical practice had found his work of an acceptable standard. It should be noted that one of the areas in which the consultant specialised involved surgical procedures that did not always have ideal outcomes.

The medical director came under scrutiny for signing the reference and the GMC decided to investigate this. They insisted on formulating a charge of professional misconduct based on the single fact of omission of any reference to suspension in the original reference.

There was no criticism with respect to unawareness of poor clinical performance or the earlier matters outside the United Kingdom.

It required a vigorous defence from the medical director's protection society and legal advisors before the GMC withdrew. This involved a lodged request for judicial review on the grounds of no jurisdiction and offences under the Human Rights Act. The emotional cost to the medical director was considerable and the media publicity most unwelcome.

This case is complex and demonstrates well the desire to apportion blame by various parties with different interests. For a Christian, it brings home sharply that the justice of this world is very different from God's justice. We are all flawed. We all make mistakes. The most important way of living for us all is to act with integrity and make judgements based on what is known at the time.

It can be argued that the General Medical Council, as a body, had an interest in focusing blame on others and avoiding too much emphasis on its own shortcomings in relation to earlier decisions to take no action.

The case became highly politicised and several groups had an interest in blaming the previous management of the Trust. The patients' group not only wished to blame the consultant but the management as well. The entire non-clinical team were gradually moved on if they had not left or retired already. This was seen to be politically astute regardless of who was at fault.

On the assumption that the charges against the consultant were fully justified one is left with a bizarre chain of events that make general conclusions very difficult to sustain. One can argue that the General Medical Council should have re-investigated the causes of removal from the register in an overseas country, regardless of inconvenience and cost, and prevented the consultant from practising in the United Kingdom if the evidence was sustained. This could have been done. The regional health authority could have rescinded their appointment, because the applicant they appointed withheld crucial information. Clinical colleagues could have raised concerns if they were aware of adverse performance. No one did so. In this case, in view of the subsequent level of patient complaint, there remains a mystery.

When something goes badly wrong we want to blame someone other than ourselves. It is certainly important to work out what went wrong in any case and that is far more important than blame. The desire to blame can distort genuine evidence and lead to inappropriate actions.

The word 'scapegoat' has a rich meaning. When Abraham prepared to sacrifice Isaac, he was saved from doing so by an animal caught in a thicket. An innocent animal was the substitute sacrifice. Why God needed any sacrifice is one of the core issues of Christianity. A goat was let loose in the wilderness on Yom

Kippur, the day of atonement. The goat carried the sins of the people after the high priest symbolically laid them on its head (Lev.16.8 10–26). Many understand Jesus as bearing the sins of the world through his death on the cross. More mundane, the death of Jesus kept the troublesome Jewish mob quiet. Rene Girard provides a searching analysis of the subject in his book *The Scapegoat.* He uses an example of the Jews being scapegoated for the Black Death in France. The Jewish people have been scapegoats throughout history. The belief that if we offer up a sacrifice for misdeeds the gods will be appeased is deeply imbedded in human culture. 'Heads roll' after enquiries and this can help appease the complainants regardless of the correct attribution of blame. 'We want blood' is as true today as it has ever been.

It is difficult to understand how one can bring charges against someone on the basis they did not refer to unfounded allegations. But of interest in this episode for the institutional Church, is how to be part of pain and stress in the work place.

One of the distinctive features of ministry in secular employment, a specialised form of ordained ministry, is that the priest is an ordinary member of the work force, exposed to the same temptations, stresses and strains as any other member of staff. That person works on the boundaries of the church, often straddling the worlds of belief and unbelief, open to insights from both.

The involvement of the Church in the world of work remains a challenge. The traditional parochial structure has some value, but requires complete re-evaluation. Decline in church attendance, relative paucity of baptisms and marriages, and with pastoral care being distant from the place of work in most cases, suggests the need for a shift towards the factory, hospital, school;

anywhere where people spend their working life. I do not refer to people with clerical collars, fulfilling the role of chaplain, but priests who work alongside their colleagues sharing the joy and pain; at the cutting point, the heart and the edge of daily working life.

When I became a tutor in practical theology in my spare time, one of my roles was to work with ordinands, teasing out the theological issues in their working world. In our course most of them retained their jobs until ordination; some went on and became ministers in secular employment; sadly, relatively few. We were exploring what has been called Kingdom theology; seeking the Kingdom of God where we spend much of our lives. It was possible to bring the world of work to the alter each Sunday, but the rest of life was not concerned with liturgies.

I recall a solicitor who was employed by the Crown Prosecution Service. He spent much of his time prosecuting disadvantaged people for minor offences. He worked in the County of Durham. We spent much time exploring how he could bring his ministry alongside these people at the margins of society; at the 'bleeding' point of a sad world. Ultimately, he gave up and chose parochial ministry. I was disappointed but understood. This was a situation that could only be worked out in situ. It was risky, potentially painful and humiliating, but God had to be there or Christianity would fail.

I think the work and writings of Simone Weil, mystic, philosopher, connects with this world. She spent time working in Auto factories, alongside others to learn what it was like to live in the world and be bruised by it. She never entered the confines of the institutional church but exemplified the need to be alongside people in the jobs they do. There can be no exceptions to this role, however challenging.

Skilled Caring

"He answered, 'Love the Lord your God with all your heart and
with all your soul and with all your strength and with all your
mind and "Love your neighbour as yourself."'
Luke 10.27

Caring is a word that finds true expression when we know that
someone is caring for us. They show concern and attention for us
as people. To some extent, at least, they have put themselves in
our position. Yet to consider caring in this way excludes many
who have influenced and sustained our lives. We concentrate on
the dramatic and the obvious and neglect the transient
interventions we barely remember or recognise.

*It had been a pleasant early summer day. They had been to
visit the North York Moors Visitor Centre. On the way down from
the hills he began to feel rather unwell. A feeling of faintness
came over him. He thought his blood sugar might be low,
because of the diabetic medication. He ate a banana but felt no
better. He drove to a nearby supermarket where they stopped and
his wife went inside to purchase a single article.*

*While she was in the shop he felt very unwell and thought he
would lose consciousness. His pulse was very irregular and he
felt faint. He lay as flat as he could and waited. When his wife
returned, they went to the casualty department of the local
hospital.*

After preliminary assessment he was admitted to the coronary care unit for observation. Although tired and somewhat apprehensive he became aware very quickly of the good humour and concern of the coronary care nurses. They combined medical knowledge, technical ability and caring.

What he failed to remember clearly was the porter who took him to the ward, the people in the laboratory whom he never saw, but were responsible for the pathology results, the lady in the pharmacy who dispensed his medication.

An example such as this is a common enough experience of many people admitted to intensive monitoring situations. The front-line staff epitomise the modern nurse and provide a clear picture of the essence of skilled care.

Caring about someone is important, but caring takes on a different dimension when it involves the exercise of professional skills. It is possible to exercise high technical skill but not care about the subject of the applied knowledge. It is unlikely that someone would bother much about his or her work if it did not bring reward, but this can vary from satisfaction in the application of knowledge, pecuniary gain and the joy of serving another. Most of us function with a combination of these motives. They are not mutually exclusive, but the absence of the caring motive makes a difference to the professional work we do. On the other hand, caring is not enough if we exercise a profession. There is an obligation to obtain and maintain knowledge and apply it appropriately.

Nurses rate very highly in the public perception of trusted professionals. Although there has been some loss in public trust of doctors, particularly hospital doctors, nursing seems to carry with it an aura of dedication and service that has survived press cynicism and public outrage.

What is it that continues to allow nursing this privileged status, regardless of whether this is a true picture of what prevails? There are plenty of stories about uncaring nurses, but this has little impact on their overall reputation.

Historically, nursing has been linked with religious orders and is a symbol of God's love expressed through human agency. Because of the connection with religion nurses have been perceived, at least implicitly, as people who give their services for little earthly reward. There is general agreement that in our secular age they remain poorly paid and their goodwill exploited by successive governments. Some might argue that the picture of the nurse as 'angel of mercy' is dependent on such a situation. If nurses were highly paid they might be open to the same degree of cynical appraisal as other professions.

It is remarkable that nurses have retained their status as icons of skilled caring. Perhaps this points to our need to admire and look up to a professional ideal that transcends our frail attempts to live our lives caring for others.

Nowadays the separation of the nursing and medical professions seems increasingly artificial. Nurses are not 'handmaids' of doctors. We should examine what the word 'nurse' stands for in relation to the word 'doctor'.

The summary of the law that Jesus taught included loving God with all our beings, mind and body and loving our neighbour in the way that we would hope to be loved. One perceived characteristic of nursing is holistic care. Nurses spend on average much more quality time with patients than doctors. They are far more likely to be present at moments of anguish and need. They often interpret what the doctor has said. Some cynics would say 'they pick up the pieces'. But nurses are not able to be there to care all the time, no one is.

In general nurses look after fewer people for longer periods of time than doctors, particularly in hospitals. However, many doctors may gain knowledge and understanding of people extended over long periods of time. This happens in general practice and those hospital specialities that are involved with chronic progressive diseases.

A possible factor that unites nursing as an ideal with some medical settings is that the greater and longer the involvement with a person, the more likely it is that holistic care is manifest. The carer is seen to be involved and interested in all aspects of a person's being. This, perhaps, is the core of the 'nursing ideal' that can transcend the profession of nursing and apply to other professions.

Yet it is unfair to assume that briefer contacts with health professionals are not caring occasions. One cannot conclude that a minor surgical procedure skilfully performed is not performed with caring motives. Surgeons working under great pressure should not be assumed to be uncaring if they are unable to spend much contact time with the people they treat.

An archbishop once gave a talk in which he discussed the idea of 'sanctified' neglect. He pointed out that in any job there is a specific area of activity that is at the core of the job. It is not possible for an archbishop to take detailed interest in individual parochial matters. He depends on others in the team to do this. Likewise, in medicine, it is impossible for people who are employed for a skill to spend too much time involved in other matters.

There is no single adequate model of caring. The moment of care may be brief or the role prolonged. It is the motive that matters. Although we know little of the historical Jesus, his active ministry appeared short. He was itinerant. It seems unlikely he spent much time in his latter period with his family. He showed 'sanctified' neglect for some aspects of life. He was concerned with the poor and needy, but he would have been limited in what he could personally do for others.

In his book *Loss and Gain* John Henry Newman has a central character, Charles Reding. He travels by train from Oxford to London and meets briefly a priest who talks with him and provides him with an introductory letter. The priest's attire is strange and foreign. Reding learns nothing of him.

"By the time they had reached Paddington and before the train had well stopped, the priest had taken his small carpet bag from under his seat, wrapped his cloak around him, stepped out of the carriage, and was walking out of sight at brisk pace." This person's background and thoughts were unknown to Reding, but he entered his life for a moment and gave great assistance.

An episode such as this resonates with the many brief interventions that are made into the lives of people as they pass through the health care system. We know little of the person who comes and takes blood, performs an electrocardiogram, supervises an X-ray, performs tests in the biochemistry laboratory, examines a pathological specimen that may dictate our future treatment. We may never see them or meet them only briefly, but they influence our lives. They may be our unrecognised or forgotten carers. What they do may be priestly. The mediaeval poem *Piers Ploughman* by William Langland is a dreamlike visionary poem, critical of corruption in the Church.

Piers, the farmer, is the true follower of Truth. He and his work are the genuine priesthood. All carers are there to try and make the world come right. Consciously or otherwise they are God's priestly agents.

Medicine and Religion – Facing up to Change?

"Every truth passes through three stages before it is recognized. In the first, it is ridiculed, in the second it is opposed, in the third it is regarded as self-evident."

Arthur Schopenhauer

It is obvious that in any doctor's working life there will be substantial movement in understanding disease processes and their management and treatment. In my own speciality of neurology there have been vast changes. Improved neurosurgical techniques have had a major impact on the treatment of cerebral aneurysms and brain tumours. Medication has become available for Parkinson's disease and there are many new drugs to treat epilepsy. The classification of muscular dystrophy and other genetic neurological disorders has changed because of molecular genetics. I have mentioned these developments previously. Research on multiple sclerosis has yielded new lines of therapeutic endeavour. The list can go on.

We know now that some practices deemed good for us in former times have the opposite effect. Perhaps the most important is the whole idea of 'bed rest'. When I qualified, people who had had heart attacks were kept in bed for several weeks. This is now known to be harmful management. Patients are out of bed after major operations in a day. Bed is now regarded as a dangerous place to be.

The basic ideal underlying all progress is the necessity of reviewing practice based on evidence available and seeking to move forward in the search for greater understanding. All this leads to new opportunities for treatment and relief of suffering. It is hard unromantic work in the main.

Although there are undoubted cultural influences in medicine, the advent of the scientific method since the Enlightenment has given science a status that isolates it, in part, from social influences. For example, if one entered a major hospital in any part of the world one would be aware of cultural differences between Britain, America, Africa and India. However, given comparable facilities, the diagnostic and treatment regimens would be similar. Modern medicine is transferable.

The future of medicine will undoubtedly involve considerable change. How this happens is not a pure scientific question. Social and political factors will interact to determine to some extent the direction taken. Molecular genetics will play an important part in the future together with the advances made in embryo research. New forms of treatment will be available. Interventions are likely to be less invasive and conventional surgery, in the long term, may become much less important. The boundaries between medical and surgical disciplines may blur. Medicine based on science will continue to evolve. Treatments and disease classification will alter with new knowledge, but this will not involve rejecting all the searching and hard graft that went before. That will be part of the narrative of the human search for greater understanding.

Christianity is imbedded in culture but some of the things we find about Christianity may seem very surprising. One soon realises that there is not a single framework one can call the Christian framework. Christianity has fragmented in a way that science has not. Before the Reformation the Western Church appeared a relatively homogeneous structure under the authority of the Pope. The rejection of papal authority was associated with a return to the Bible as the source of Christian doctrine and new denominations were spawned claiming their own truths. Denominational rivalry flourished and the Church fragmented and remains so to this day.

The Enlightenment further undermined the whole idea of divine authority in favour of personal development and the search for scientific truth. Earlier, Galileo and Copernicus had demonstrated that 'the heavens' were not separate; our world was just a small planet along with many others. Our world was not the centre of the universe. However, these paradigm shifts in understanding did not change the Church as much as one would expect. The biggest shake-up came with the work of Darwin on evolution in the nineteenth century. People began to realise that the Earth was of great age and had evolved over aeons of time. Human life and language had emerged gradually from earlier life forms. The Earth and all in it was not created in six days.

Inevitably, this had a major impact on Christianity that remains unresolved. Acceptance of the need to change has been slow and inadequate. Some have found it impossible to accept such new knowledge and hang on to a creationist picture of the world. Broadly, one could say that Christianity has become more fragmented within its denominational splits. It is insufficient to use terms such as liberal and conservative to describe the various manifestations of Christianity. There are splits that affect several features of the Christian religion. There is a difference between the Western world and Christianity in Africa and other developing nations. But in the West, there are several developing traditions that threaten to tear asunder the fragile veneer of unity, within, for example, Anglicanism. There are those who adhere to the Bible as understood by them as the supreme authority on all matters and the absolute divine word of God. Others take a more liberal approach to scripture but hold on to the essential dogmatic framework enshrined in the historic creeds, the divine status of Jesus and the literal truth of the bodily resurrection. A further group, exemplified by the Jesus seminar in the USA and the 'Sea of Faith' movement follow the path of progressive Christianity, questioning much of the so called 'factual' basis of the religion and concentrating on the mythological nature of Christian narrative. This latter group most closely follows the basic tenet of the search for scientific truth, that nothing is beyond questioning or challenge and the Christian faith has no special status that protects it from this type of enquiry. However, even in this group, as one might expect in the scientific community, there are layers of opinion; from the recognition of a theistic concept of God to abolition of God altogether. God is then the summit of all that is best in human aspirations and endeavours but not an entity beyond us.

My own view of science is that it is deeply mysterious and rational at the same time. It is quite possible to embrace a 'spiritual' understanding of creation while being completely committed to scientific exploration. Is this possible to achieve with religion? I believe it is, but radical change is required, particularly with dogmatic religions such as Christianity.

One of the 'boasts' of Christianity is its unchanging status. The Bible represents a core of unchanging divine truth. Doctrine was developed by the early Church Fathers and is just as relevant today as it was then. However, if one examines early Christian literature it is evident that there was great intellectual debate about the nature of Jesus, the Resurrection and authority within the Church. Christian debate was stifled in part by the politicisation of the Faith under Constantine. It suited the Roman World of that time to have a faith with clear cut authority lines and thus heterodox beliefs were anathematised and suppressed.

I am not at all sure that orthodox Christianity will survive long term in the West as a major institution without creative exploration of Christian myths in the light of modern knowledge. There will be those who continue to hold traditional beliefs, but the younger generation will seek a more open spirituality. Most of my own children have found orthodox Christianity a problem. They see it as out of step with the modern world; disengaged from reality, but at the same time attempting to be trendy, and even embracing managerial culture. The Bishop as chief executive officer is an awful prospect. The influence of the Church is diminishing and disestablishment in the United Kingdom might reduce its impact further. It is not possible to predict with any certainty whether the Church hierarchy will gradually encourage theological diversity explicitly. Overall, those who attend Anglican Churches in the United Kingdom are theologically naive. However, many of them are open to new ways of looking at Christianity. There may well be pockets of 'orthodoxy', but we have moved into a world full of uncertainty and the clinging to reassuring old certainties is an illusion. The world is becoming ready for bold spiritual explorers, who do not ignore the traditions and figures of the past, but continue in the spirit of science to search for truth and understanding. In my view the search for God can unite people, but the figure of Jesus, or rather some Christian claims about Jesus, can divide the world

That may be thought to be a terrible attack on the fiduciary framework that generations have lived by. It is entirely natural to defend traditional views. But that does not make them 'right'.

Whether we can develop a 'new' spirituality based on past insights and a present and future revelation is the ultimate challenge for institutional religion and for us all. Science beckons the way. We must move from false certainty and seek release to search for the Divine.

Despite a fear that Christianity would collapse if we re-evaluated Jesus, there is no good evidence that I know of that supports this notion. The traditional Church might suffer but it is time for Christianity to move beyond institutions. True Christianity has never been defined by dogma and structures.

Yet, I see no reason why our ancient liturgies need to be abandoned entirely. For many they remain a rich source of metaphor and myth that lead us to the heart of the Divine. They are not the mystery but we are helped to focus our hearts and minds. If this was made much clearer to seekers after God or the mystery of 'Being' many would feel a great sense of relief.

I have referred to the demise of traditional Christianity; the version that emphasises sin, atonement and a literal interpretation of doctrines such as the virgin birth. Most, if not all, great Christian doctrines can be helpful in a metaphorical or mythological sense, but it is no longer tenable to insist that they have the status of a scientific proof. I do not foresee radical change for many generations, particularly in developing countries, but the call for change has always been there.

Through a Glass Darkly

"For now we see only a reflection as in a mirror; then we shall see face to face. Now I know in part; then I shall know fully, even as I am fully known."
I Corinthians 13.12

Existential philosophy has no answers for us about why we are here. We can know nothing about the fundamental issues of existence. Life is either mysterious or fundamentally meaningless. The only meaning that can be obtained is through our own engagement as 'beings' in the world. There is no transcendent reality. If one accepts the brutal analysis of secular existentialism one is content to accept this limitation and the desire to know more is absent. Yet many of us want to know 'Being' or the source of our existence. Yet it has seemed to me impossible to know fully anything or anyone in this world and we have to rely on the possibility, but only the possibility, of enlightenment beyond this life. The problem of knowing anything beyond the surface facts is something that may spur us in our search. But in the end, we may conclude that all we know is how little we know, and therefore reluctant to be too opinionated.

The practice of medicine is increasingly founded in scientific knowledge. The knowledge base changes but the principal of applying new knowledge to medicine does not. Yet there is much more to medical practice than science. Science may provide a certain kind of knowledge, but decision making is based on more than knowledge. Whatever the discipline we only know 'in part'.

For many years, I have been interested in the variation in the clinical skill of individual practitioners. This is not necessarily based on differences in knowledge or scientific ability. It seems to depend on the ability to look below the surface of any transaction. To some extent this could be equated with the concept of sound judgement but it is more than that.

In the introduction to these essays and elsewhere, I have referred to the work of Proust and his final novel *Time Regained*. Proust was convinced that it is quite possible to go through the narrative of life without ever approaching the depths of 'being'. We may never have a glimpse of the fullness of knowing, but some people have brief insights. That may seem a very elitist view and an insult to the millions who struggle for survival and who have no time for deep thought. But I think what Proust is describing is at least partly a gift and is independent of the length of time one spends thinking or analysing. Insight often comes as a surprise. It is perhaps an outcome of intuitive behaviour. Intuition linked with scientific knowledge helps one to be a 'good doctor'.

I am not sure what the neurological basis for intuition is. We must be very careful when we try to explain everything through an analysis of brain function and anatomy. Roger Penrose, the eminent scientist, is concerned about the nature of truth. He questions how we judge what is true or untrue about creation. He suggests, very unusually for a mathematician, that perhaps intuition or instinct might be relevant in approaching the truth of propositions.

In the late 1960s I was trying to make ends meet by doing some emergency night calls while doing my daytime job as a senior registrar in neurology. There were no mobile telephones in those days, so I would start out in my own car with the first call, and afterwards telephone from a box to obtain the next visit. On one stormy winter night, I was called to a tower block in West Newcastle. A young child was screaming on arrival at the top of the block. A general practitioner had visited earlier in the day and diagnosed a viral infection. The child was conscious and there were no convincing localizing signs. The tonsils looked a little red. What should I make of it all? I was tired and the child's family was in chaos. There was a powerful feeling that I should just leave it to the morning. It was very difficult to get admissions for uncertain diagnoses at that time of year. But something told me that this child had meningitis. I went and made a telephone call to the local hospital; the flat had no telephone. I rang the nearest hospital and got a negative response and then tried my own. I was about to be refused again when I pulled rank and made it quite clear that as I had considerable neurological knowledge the duty doctor had better not turn me down. I told him he could berate me in the morning if I was wrong. I was far from sure of myself; a dingy poorly-lit flat is a far cry from the hospital ward. The next day I was informed that the child had *haemophilus influenzae* meningitis, a very dangerous condition. My instincts and intuition had been correct. I breathed a great sigh of relief.

My intuitive judgment concerning the child was based on my training and knowledge base. Sound clinical 'hunches' are a very useful short cut to diagnosis. In my view, the same intuition has an important role in examining the possibilities of religious truth. A knowledge base of a faith may combine with the level of knowledge one has about everything else to bring about intuitive judgments concerning 'religious truth'. This has led many people to conclude that aspects of Christianity need re-evaluating.

A prime example of this is the intuition that there is something wrong about understanding Christianity as an exclusive faith that is superior to all others. It is possible to know a great deal about Christianity, but be unable to intuit 'truth' that lies beyond the framework one lives by. This prevents contact with anything like a comprehensive picture of reality. The instinct of someone who is aware of the diversity of world cultures may well be to conclude that all doctrines of exclusion and particularity are suspect. The words 'believing in' or 'knowing' are greatly overused. It is better to seek rather than to believe in things. Beliefs can and do change during our lives. Earlier on in this book, I recalled the experience during depression that God *is*. That was accompanied by no assurance about doctrine at all. It seemed at the time completely irrelevant. For me, that moment was saying that beyond all formal religion there is God. Our doctrines, whatever our faiths, are only pointers to God. It is not necessary to abandon traditional frameworks, but they are not absolutes and they need to be used creatively.

I have referred to difficulties knowing why there is evil in the world; why we suffer; the problem of projecting our own concepts of 'loving' on to God. Any explanations inevitably fail. We are challenged to provide these answers but they do not satisfy; they become convoluted, lacking elegance. Instinct tells us that we would be much better off accepting our lack of knowledge and understanding. If one considers that there is no 'loving' God, there is no problem anyway. Our only way of looking at the various aspects of love is through human experience. Christianity has taken the figure of Jesus as a teacher of wisdom; a person spirit filled; an example of a loving person and a counter-culture figure. In our imaginations, we may feel he is like God or even part of the Godhead.

Our attempts to know things may lead to overelaboration. Although we may warm to the Trinitarian concept of the Godhead, it seems convoluted rather than comprehensive, simplistic rather than satisfying. Bede Griffiths, mentioned elsewhere, tried to explore the Trinity in the core of Hinduism. He may have been mistaken. Christians have attempted to incorporate Christian doctrines into other religions, but I think they fail. I would prefer to see each religion as a partial contribution to knowledge of the Divine but not capable of being fused. We may not feel comfortable excluding other incarnate figures with a similar message to Jesus. The existence of the many salvific figures in religion emphasise our partial knowledge. For the Hindu, Krishna represents a Christlike figure and there are other avatars of Vishnu that allow a more inclusive picture of incarnation. The Buddha was a similar figure to Jesus. He sought a path that gave release from attachment, the cause of all suffering (dukkha). In Buddhist mythology, he left family to follow a path of seeking. There is an element of separation in extreme forms of discipleship in many religions. Mohammed was a great prophet who appeared in a cultural setting in the deserts of Arabia. Islamic theology does not seek to give divine status to him. Islam honours Jesus but does not seek to give him or any prophet divine status. However, sects within Islam believe that there will be another caliph in the direct line of Mohammed at some time in the future. Some Jews look for a messiah who is to come. All these images and myths point to the inadequacy of knowledge.

Despite this, all these faiths are serious attempts to come to terms with life on Earth and give meaning to existence. But they are *attempts* and true knowledge of the Divine or God or any other word we wish to apply to the ground of our being lies beyond any religion. Any religion is an uncertain pathway, a search for knowledge. There is nothing inappropriate about following an established path. It is an essential element to any spiritual journey. There is no real problem in being persuaded that the path one has taken is appropriate for oneself in the cultural setting one belongs to. However, extremism and intolerance in any religion has nothing to do with any genuine spiritual journey and should be condemned without hesitation. They reflect a spurious certainty.

Sadly, this does not happen and extremists can flourish, without religious leaders speaking clearly against them. Christianity is no exception. If I was born in Myanmar, I would expect to be a Buddhist and would have no need to change my faith. The world contains many cultures and many stages of understanding of the place of religion in daily life. It seems very unlikely that we can expect uniformity in religious belief and expression in the foreseeable future. As I see it the only hope is for more understanding of the relative nature of the formularies within religious structures and our common purpose in exploring the ultimate source of our being.

In medical science, one may choose a certain path to follow in terms of research and development. This can become all-consuming and occupy much thinking time. However, the scientist will not believe that his/her corner of activity is anything other than a small part of the whole. For those who seek to know God the challenge is irresistible; it has the same grip on people as any scientific journey. Whether the human brain has the design or capacity for either form of 'knowing' is another matter altogether.

From Certainty to Mystery

"In human life, you will find players of religion until the knowledge and proficiency in religion will be cleansed from all superstitions, and will be purified and perfected by the enlightenment of real science."
Kemal Ataturk

"I like the scientific spirit—the holding off, the being sure but not too sure, the willingness to surrender ideas when the evidence is against them: this is ultimately fine—it always keeps the way beyond open—always gives life, thought, affection, the whole man, a chance to try over again after a mistake—after a wrong guess."
Walt Whitman, Walt Whitman's Camden Conversations

This book bears the title at the head of this chapter. It is shorthand for describing the growing awareness in my life that we can be certain about very little. I have experienced this through medicine, religion and personal disability. Yet it is obvious that my experience differs from others. I do not seek primarily to change minds and within certain limits I am not concerned whether people want to believe in things literally that I am unable to accept. I do protest that all religions must learn to absorb differing views and that those who lead them become more creative in doctrinal understanding and expression. There is no room for rigid interpretation of historical doctrines that disallows questioning and mystery. What follows is a summary of my thoughts; many of them expressed elsewhere. Repetition is inevitable traveling along the circle of life!

I was staying with a friend in Brisbane and we got to discussing going to church and her vision of Christianity. She loved services and appreciated the mystery and beauty of liturgy. Church provided for her a gateway to the world of otherness. She did not have orthodox beliefs. Doctrines were stories; human attempts to classify and explain. They could not be believed literally and perhaps some were simply unhelpful. The Bible was literature like any other literature. It had to be understood as such and contained good things and bad. It was not a reliable guide and certainly not a textbook of ethics. This view is a common one. I have encountered it repeatedly throughout my working life. There is every reason to listen to it. The Church should respond by listening rather than hoping that people will be persuaded to adopt positions that life has already caused them to abandon.

The word 'certainty' may be misunderstood and may mean different things in differing contexts. In the first chapter, I described how as a young boy I prayed to be cured of an eye problem. The basis for such a prayer may have been the words "Ask and it will be given unto you, seek and you will find." Somehow, it did not work. At best, it was a serious misunderstanding of Christian scripture, at worst the whole idea of religion needed to be abandoned. The fact that I did not and have not abandoned my spiritual journey, despite many temptations to do so, is at the heart of this book. I have concluded that there is no need for the many certainties that we cling to and that much of our thinking is governed by fear of uncertainty and our personal extinction.

I have already described my early experience of highly conservative evangelical Christianity, but I repeat a version of it here as it is necessary for picturing the movements I have made.

The Christianity I was born into was Bible based. Holy Scripture was the guide to all things. The Bible was essentially inerrant and could be relied upon absolutely. There was only one interpretation of the Bible and that was the one that existed in the religious setting I grew up in. Sin was real, a personal devil was real. Repentance meant turning one's own back on a life of sin and accepting Jesus Christ as one's saviour. This conferred on one salvation, an immediate transaction. This salvation was permanent. It was obtained through the atonement that was explained as the substitutionary death of Jesus on the Cross for the sins of the whole world. He rose from the dead and was in heaven with God. He would come to Earth again. There would be a major battle at Armageddon and Jesus would reign on earth for a thousand years. Then there would be the end of time. The reward that came with salvation was eternal life and that meant that after death one would rise from the dead and live for ever in heaven in direct continuity with one's previous self.

Jesus was the only Son of God. He was born by the Holy Spirit of a pure virgin. He knew he was the Son of God while on earth and performed many miracles.

The Sabbath or Sunday for the Christian was holy. One should read the Bible and go to Church. Reading other books, playing games, going shopping or having a jolly good time was discouraged. One should study the Bible and learn as much of it as possible. There was a responsibility to speak to others about

Jesus. A high calling was to go to the mission field overseas to convert other people to Christianity. Christianity was the only true religion and the conservative fundamentalist version was the only proper one. Many people who called themselves Christians were not and were as 'lost' as any pagan. The Pope was anti-Christ and featured in the book of Revelation.

This brief snapshot of my early religious background may seem a crude caricature of a certain form of evangelical Christianity, but it is as I remember it. In fact, I was not unhappy and enjoyed Sundays with all my friends when I was not at school. We would go to church morning, afternoon and evening. In the afternoon, we had pastor's class and tea at church. There was often an open-air service on the promenade after the church service. We would take part and then go on to a coffee bar. Sometimes we would move to a house setting and have a young person's speaker.

It was a world of certainty; everything was laid out for one. The word 'doubt' was not in the vocabulary. There was very strong pressure to toe the 'party line' and seem as sure and happy as everyone else was about this religious structure. Of course, the word faith is not compatible with certainty, but it is the certainty that I remember and the difficulty I had in being certain.. My own temperament did not sit easily with this fundamentalist world view. Despite the indoctrination I received it never succeeded deep down in convincing me. I had an enquiring mind and found neat solutions difficult. I enjoyed poetry from an early age and found boring extemporary prayers lacking in beauty.

One quotation at the beginning of this chapter is from Kemal Ataturk, the founder of modern Turkey following the fall of the Ottoman Empire, and it expresses his thoughts about the religion of Islam. I hasten to add that I intend no attack on Islam but have used the quotation to draw attention to a kind of religious extremism that excludes other interpretations or variations. Walt Whitman expresses the wonder of science, the openness of seeking, the acceptability of error. I presume Ataturk would have agreed with him. I am not referring to what might be termed 'simpler' forms of religious devotion. 'Simple', but at the same time mature faith is encountered in those who are willing to acknowledge the mystery of being in a spirit of openness, while being content to live out their faith within the structures they have inherited. I have encountered this most often in rural communities. Beyond this, the world is full of superstition and a vast variety of religious practices. Providing they are harmless to others and do not involve exclusive claims there is little problem with them. Many may think that it is essential that we draw all cultures into 'the modern world' and Mustafa Kemal may well have thought this, but it is not what I am getting at. Dangerous extremism is the issue. It may or may not be associated with physical violence but there are aspects of extremism that damage others in all great religions, including Christianity. In my own case, I think that most of us growing up at that time did not connect with the extremist views that were spoken in pulpits from time to time. In some way, we separated ourselves from the words we heard. It was only the hierarchy that formed the hard religious core of bigotry and exclusivism. At the time, I was unable to express doubts because of fear of being cast out from my social circle, but time and fresh pastures altered that.

Science or more particularly medical science has been a major influence on my life; not only science, but the practice of medical neurology. I was exposed to the vastness yet limitation of the human scientific knowledge base, and the necessity for change, to progress and understand disease better. There was no resting on laurels in science, no revelation that could not be improved upon, no corpus of doctrine that could not be changed. All there was, amounted to the search for truth and better understanding. This meant that in theory one could spend one's life up a blind alley looking in the wrong place for the answer to a problem. My own brief period of direct laboratory research was into multiple sclerosis. We were chipping away at something important but our own individual contributions seemed nothing. It soon seemed to me that although science sought answers, and that good science was honest, there were distasteful aspects of science that were governed by deep ambition, dishonesty and the search for quick results. However, at its best there was a deep sense of mystery and awe at the heart of the enterprise.

Cosmology, including the search for life beyond the Earth, exposes the limitations of a faith that reduces God to an entity concerned with one part of the cosmos. The vastness of the universe expands our sense of mystery. It has always seemed to me that even if we could explain everything, we would still be left with a core mystery.

We now know a great deal more about brain structure and function than when I qualified. The emergent quality of mind remains a marvel to those with a capacity for a sense of wonder. The evidence is that we are not divided people with distinct and separate spirits or souls. This need not destroy any sense of mystery or belief in God. However, it does have major bearing on some doctrinal certainties.

My initial religious framework was without mystery. It was wordy, conceptual; in retrospect, without any charm. Although I escaped it eventually, I had to allow myself to let go of many things and realise that life and our attempts to answer the great questions of existence cannot be reduced to systematic frameworks, however tempting. They provide false reassurance.

At medical school, I had a close friend we will call Arthur. We shared a flat together and we were both leading members of the Christian Union. We had similar religious upbringings and both became eventually consultant physicians within our own specialties. Meeting some years later we compared notes. Arthur had completely abandoned Christianity, describing it in his forthright way as nonsense. He had been quite an establishment figure in evangelical circles and this was a major turnaround. Although he never told me the reasons, I assumed that he could no longer reconcile Christian doctrine with life experience. He was therefore honest and I admire him for it. The framework he started with was rigid. For him there was no room for modification. It was all or nothing. By this stage I had many doubts, but saw no reason to abandon my Christian framework. I was actively thinking about alternative expressions of Christianity within which I would feel more comfortable.

My main initial preoccupation was with the various doctrines that I had been taught. These are summarized in the ancient creeds. In Anglicanism the Nicene Creed is said each Sunday during the Eucharist. The Apostles Creed is said at Matins and Evensong. Christian orthodoxy is spelt out in inaccessible language in the Nicene Creed. This creed is an inadequate attempt to rationalise the experience of those who embraced the emerging Christian faith. To some it may provide a sense of mystery. To others, the creeds are a distraction, attempting to confine that which cannot be defined. When I was training for ordination our principal would draw a line on the floor and ask us to stand on it according to our position on the content of the Nicene Creed. At one end there were those who fully accepted it and at the other end those who rejected it completely. Many took the middle ground. The exercise demonstrated that any creed is not the last word on Christianity. Perhaps, we need to be released from them to re-explore without prescription.

One of the most difficult credal statement is the one about Jesus as being uncreated, begotten of the Father. This means that there was no point at which Jesus the Son of God 'was not'. This was an issue that separated Arius and Athanasius, both from Alexandria. Arius was anethamatised for his failure to accept some of the detail, as he insisted that Jesus was in some sense created. This kind of technical disagreement exposes the folly of reducing theological statements to exclusive definitions.

I have mentioned other doctrines previously; the virgin birth is unsustainable as an account of true human nature; miracles belonged to their day but cannot be translated to the modern world; the Resurrection can be understood as literal or metaphorical; the atonement may be an example of the willingness to sacrifice one's life for a cause, but the idea that God required Jesus' death as a price or payment for the sins of all people is another matter altogether. I have admired the work Geza Vermes, the Jewish theologian, who was a Roman Catholic monk, before reverting to Judaism. He had a Jewish friend, John Winter, another exile from persecution, who wrote a little known book *On the Trial of Jesus.* Vermes concludes his book on *The Resurrection* with a quotation from Winter. I have found this to encapsulate the mystery of following Jesus. "Sentence was passed and Jesus was led away. Crucified, dead and buried, he yet rose in the hearts of his disciples who had loved him and felt he was near. Tried by the world, condemned by authority, buried by the Churches that profess his name, he is rising again, today and tomorrow, in the hearts of people who love him and feel he is near." That is the mystery of Jesus and it lies beyond certainty and formulations.

What is religion for? For me, the primary purpose of religion is worship of the mystery of our existence and an aid to living a life that is less self-centered than it might have been. In worship, we seek to be in contact with God through ritual and any other helpful parts of liturgy that take us beyond ourselves and the temporal world. Religion is about searching for the ultimate source of our being, the 'Other' that touches our lives. It seems to me that worship and seeking God, or whatever name we wish to use, gives rise to secondary outcomes that enhance our lives; qualities such as the capacity to love, to serve. These lead to salvation or release from ourselves towards true life. Eternal qualities enter the mundane world of temporary phenomena.

After my exposure to Indian culture and history I found it quite impossible to consider Christianity as the only true religion or Jesus as the only vehicle of God's wisdom and salvation. Natural common sense tells one that if there is a god, he is not to be revealed absolutely at one time and in one cultural setting and in one unique individual. We may have a natural sense of alienation when we meet a culture radically different to our own for the first time, but unfamiliarity is not a good reason for rejecting differing cultures and religions.

I may have appeared extremely negative about doctrines such as the Resurrection, Atonement and Incarnation, but they may be sources of inspiration for us. We can look at Resurrection as something entirely positive and an essential goal in a spiritual journey, dwelling on the mystery expressed so eloquently by Paul Winter. Jesus spoke clearly about losing life and finding it and the Buddha did the same. These words can speak a great deal to us about true life on this Earth, removed from desire and selfishness, and orientated towards service and meeting the needs of others. That for me is true resurrection. Similarly, the Atonement need not be some strange transaction almost like a chemical reaction. Atonement and the Cross speak of sacrificial living. Jesus is an exemplar for all of us and one who could follow his vision to the end with integrity. He is a universal figure that challenges us. That might not have been the case, but our cultural history has determined that his influence and power remain today. As a young person, I was inspired by Albert Schweitzer. He was a man of his age and a notable missionary and scholar. He encapsulated for me the mystery of following Jesus as he described it at the end of his book – *The Quest for the Historical Jesus.* Jesus is a remote mysterious figure standing beside the Sea of Galilee; he summons people to follow him. We should respond, if we are called, in a manner appropriate to our times and dispositions. There is no master plan, no detailed guide.

We may eventually arrive at a place of knowing everything and knowing nothing; a state of silence and complete simplicity. There are no questions to answer and none to ask. Our vision is unlimited, and our abode is both totally full and completely empty. We are beyond anxiety, and we believe everything and nothing. There are no promises, no hope. There is stillness, life and no life. We have arrived at this limitless pool down a long river with many tributaries. We have travelled back and forth, returned and started again. On our arrival, there is no need for satisfaction and there is no way back. We have passed beyond mystery.

Postscript

Christianity has been an important framework for me. It has enabled me to explore human spirituality through a structure that has promoted study, reflection and encouraged a way of life centered on an attempt to follow Jesus. During my life, I have had to let go many of the certainties about dogmatic religious belief as part of a quest to live an integrated existence. I have moved beyond the formal structures that defined what I should or should not believe until the word 'belief' has seemed unsuitable in the context of a spiritual journey. Many people would affirm the adage that as one ages there is a tendency to believe more and more about less and less.

A global perspective seems essential in evaluating religious claims because the spiritual and cultural histories of this diverse world demand an open and sympathetic evaluation. Religious exclusivity continues to exist but is difficult to sustain if one listens to the spiritual masters from different but overlapping explorations of the significance of earthly existence.

Whatever name one gives to God or the source of all, it is possible with integrity to continue to believe that beyond the discoveries of science there lies a spiritual reality that is present but beyond comprehension. Science does not explain our existence. Some of the 'How' questions may be answered but the 'Why' question continues to haunt us. It is possible to conclude that this question should not be asked, but the fact that we seek, is a human trait despite no definitive conclusions. The many prophets and gods that occupy religious tradition may provide us with moments of illumination, but no prophet and no defined god provides an exclusive map of what to believe or how to live.

Christianity was born in the Roman-Hellenist world and much influenced by Greek thought and culture. Constantine established Christianity as the official religion of the Roman Empire. Prior to this from around 330 BCE, with the conquests of Alexander the Great, Hellenism dominated the known world. The pantheon of the ancient gods shitted to allow greater individual forms of worship. Gods and goddesses such as Isis, Demeter, Mithras and Dionysus became connected with mystery cults. Alexandria in Egypt became a melting pot for creative religious thinking. Philo, the Jewish philosopher, introduced allegorical interpretation and Platonic ideas into Judaism. Gnosticism, widely regarded as a Christian heresy and a complex mixture of world views, flourished in the second and third centuries CE, and Gnostics such as Basiledes and Valentinus produced complex theological variants of Christianity. A body of writing known as the Corpus Hermeticum or the Hermetica originated in the region of Alexandria in the late first, second and third centuries. Some of the ideas about the nature of God, imbued with a mixture of Stoic and Platonic thought found in the Hermetica and the writings of Basiledes and Valentinus, may be present in the Gospel of John.

This period of several hundred years was a time of great change. Thinkers were attempting to answer fundamental questions concerning: What am I, where do I come from, what is my destiny and how should I live? The eventual establishment of orthodox Christianity under Constantine's conquests, and insistence on a uniform version of the new religion, culminated in the historic creeds, starting in Nicaea in 325 CE. This provided an all-embracing framework for people to live by that dominated the Western World and the Eastern Orthodox Churches for centuries. The rise of science and the overthrow of the dominating influence of Aristotle on Christian theology, started in the seventeenth century with Descartes. Since that time the expanse of human knowledge about the world and about ourselves as beings in the world has precipitated a further historic period of human uncertainty. This has been the predominant feature of life in the 'Western' world. Cultures more distant from the Enlightenment have partially escaped this.

It is my view that we remain in that period. Despite the apparent triumph of science, we are unsure of our place in the universe and the great questions of existence continue to concern those who pause to reflect. World wars have been part of the process that has seen the erosion of systematic theologies and the advent of the fragmentation associated with modernism and post-modernism. *The Waste Land* by TS Eliot exemplified the feeling of futility that followed the First World War. The rise of analytical philosophy, rather than the all-embracing approach of traditional metaphysics, pointed to a reluctance to accept systematic approaches to the fundamental issues of existence. Secular Existentialism has provided an earthy approach to the practicalities of the human predicament, developed in one form by Jean Paul Sartre, and originating in Continental Europe after the Second World War.

The gradual decline in church attendance is a symptom of dissatisfaction with neat answers to the basic problems of existence. There may be other factors at the root of the decline in church membership, but the dogma of Christian orthodoxy prevents many from any involvement with institutional religion. Sociological studies suggest that belief in God, or an ultimate source of Being, has not declined in the same way; but there is a preference to pursue a spiritual quest on an individual basis unhampered by dogmatic expectation. Globalisation has required all religions to reassess any exclusivity they claim, and this has been an important but neglected problem for Christianity and Christology. The future of Christianity is difficult to predict and it continues to flourish in some developing countries, frequently in a conservative form. In the West, the future surely lies in an exploratory quest for enlightenment, open to change and reassessment. Paradoxically, religious frameworks retain value providing their relativity and cultural settings are recognised. Religious pluralism does not undermine the pilgrim quest but enhances it. The recognition that most if not all religions are united by an awareness that there is an ultimate source of all being, regardless of name, should be at the heart of any future for religion. It is the claims of the individual saviours and prophets of these faiths that may divide people.

During the modern era, science has developed at an astonishing pace. The twentieth and twenty-first centuries have witnessed rapid increases in life expectancy through social and medical advances. An increase in genetic knowledge is heralding an era of individualised medicine in the management of disease. We are actively pursuing the search for life elsewhere in the Cosmos. The spirit of enquiry that has led to scientific progress is an example of the spirit that is needed in any religious quest or pilgrimage. The word 'openness' is one way of expressing this attitude to life. Another word of importance is 'imagination'. My third word would be 'integrity'. No one should build a concrete wall around their religious beliefs or searches. Interaction across all aspects of life is essential to any understanding of why we are here and how we should live.

Science does not make religion irrelevant. The framework of any religion continues to help us explore the spiritual territory that lies beyond the empirical enquiries of science. Yet ultimately that framework falls away, or has served its purpose, as we pass beyond its limits to embrace a greater reality.

Some Suggested Reading

Karen Armstrong: *The Battle for God.* London. Harper Collins 2000.

Maurice Wiles: *God's Action in the World.* London SCM 1986.

Peter Baelz: *Does God Answer Prayer* Dartman Longman and Todd 1982.

Peter Baelz: *Prayer and Providence – a background study* Hulsean lectures SCM 1986.

Peter Bishop: *Written on the Flyleaf – Christian Faith in the light of other Faiths.* London, Epworth 1998.

Alan Race, *Christianity and Other Faiths*, London. SCM. 1983.

Helen Oppenheimer *Looking before and After*, London, Collins Fount 1988.

Gaza Vermes *Jesus the Jew London* SCM 2000.

Harold S Kushner: *When Bad Things Happen to Good People* Anchor Books, New York. New York 2004.

Arthur Peacocke: *Creation and the World of Science – The Reshaping of Belief.* Oxford University Press Oxford and New York 2004.

John Hick: *Death and Eternal Life* Westminster John Knox Press 1996

John Dominic Crossan and NT Wright: *The Resurrection of Jesus,* Augsburg Press, Minneapolis, USA 2006.

Geza Vermes: *The Resurrection,* Penguin Books, London and New York 2008.

Harry Williams: *True Resurrection*, Holt, Rinehart and Winstan, 1972.

Mary Warnock: *Do Human Cells have Rights?* Bioethics 1987 January; 1 (1): 1–14.

Maurice O'C. Drury: *The Danger of Words (Wittgenstein studies)* Thoemmes Continuum; 2nd revised edition 1996.

The Upanishads: translated by John Mascaro by Penguin books London 1965.

Rig Veda: translated RTH Griffith and JL Shastri Motilal Banarsidaas 1995.

Rene Girard: *The Scapegoat* translated by Yvonne Freccaro the John Hopkins University Press Baltimore 1986.

Marcus Borg: *Convictions – How I Learned what matters most* HarperOne 2014.

Marvin Meyer (Editor*) The Nag Hammadi Scriptures: The Revised and Updated Translation of Sacred Gnostic Texts Complete in One Volume Harper Collins 2009.*